Table Of Contents

Introduction

Since November 2014, I have helped more than 30,000 people online and locally in Las Vegas find new ways to improve their health with plant based solutions. My objective was simple, I was going to transform their health from ordinary to extraordinary. I wanted to help people break free the physical boundaries and limits that their bodies had placed on them as time became less on their side.

Ever since my own my mom got triple bypass surgery when I was 14 years old, I've been passionate about helping people not go down the same path as her. This means focusing on eating more live and whole foods, increasing energy levels naturally, reducing the visible signs of aging, and minimizing the amount of cellulite on the body.

This all starts with what we eat and I realize that recipes don't come with a cape and aren't going to save the day, but they are a step in the right direction towards reaching your ideal body weight by having healthier options. My hope is that you see how quick and easy these foods are to make once you get the hang of things and incorporate them into your life as a part of a more whole foods lifestyle.

The infographics, recipes, and supplements in this book are just the tip of the iceberg and there's plenty of more where this came from but I wanted to give you some food for thought and to show you why you matter so much to me!

- Lance McGowan

Problem #1: Stress

Did you know? *75-90% of all doctor visits in the U.S. are for stress related ailments.*

Free radicals can damage cellular DNA, mitochondria, and other critical cell structures

Short-term cellular damage can trigger a defensive response in cells

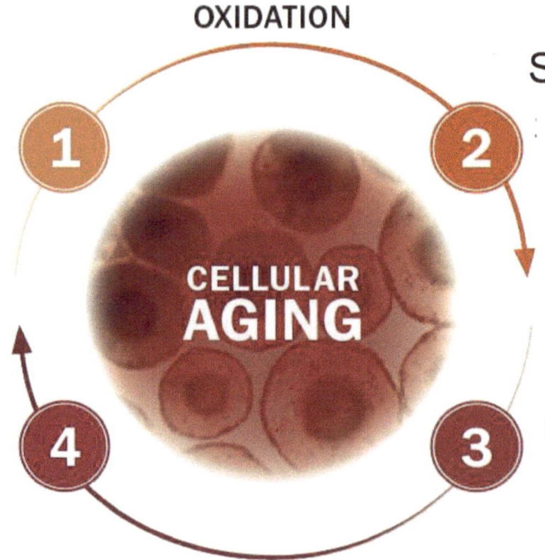

Damaged cells can lead to unhealthy aging

Cells, tissues, and organs become more prone to oxidative stressors

Natural Solutions

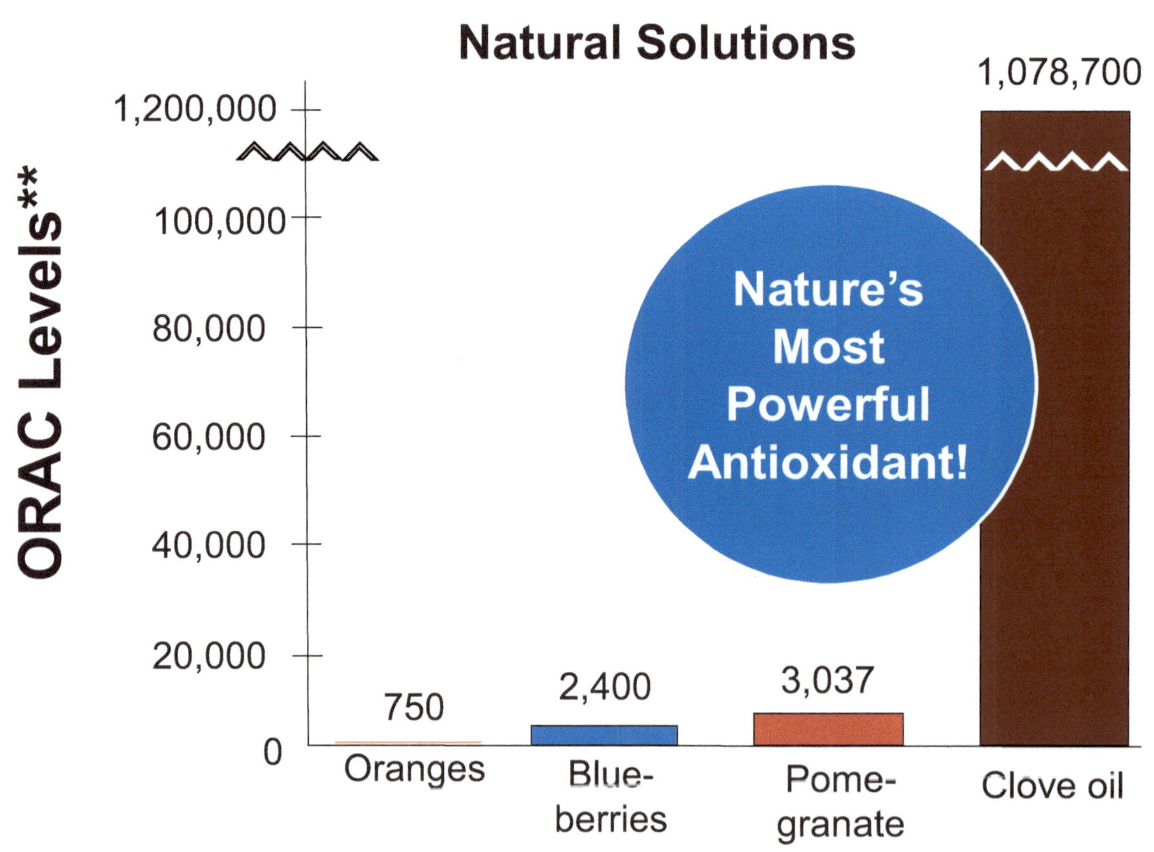

*Source: The essential life, 2015

**Source: Using God's Medicine for the Abundant Life, 2015

**Oxygen radical absorbance capacity (ORAC) is a method of measuring antioxidant capacities in biological samples 4

Problem #2: Sleep

- Worsening sleep quality and sleep duration are associated with a greater build up of amyloid beta (proteins) in the brain

- The failure of the brain to keep it's house clean by clearing away waste like amyloid beta, may contribute to the development of conditions like Alzheimer's.

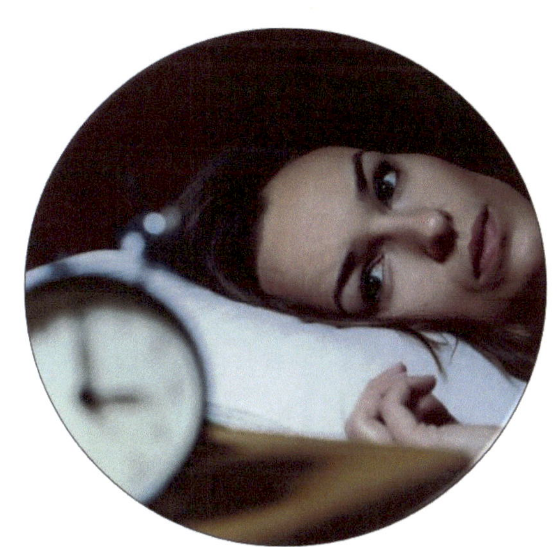

Natural Solutions

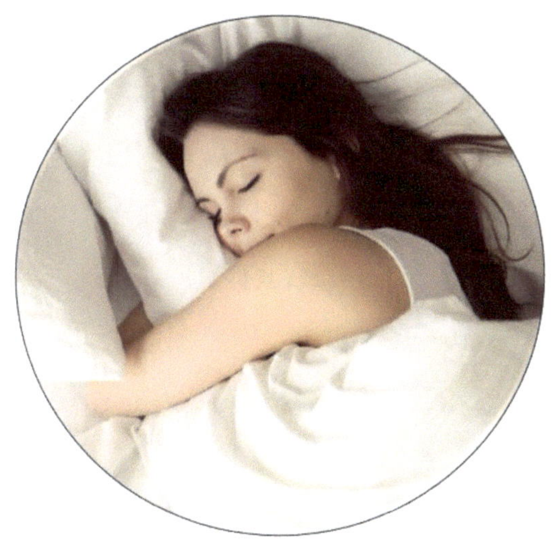

1.) Develop a **nightly routine** and get 7-9 hours of sleep (e.g. writing down thoughts in a planner to help calm the mind chatter)

2.) **Trace minerals**: Every function in the body needs minerals, but almost everyone is nutrient deficient. Fulvic acid is most bioavailable form of minerals (rocks are low)

3.) Lavender, marjoram, roman chamomile

Problem #3: Digestion

Did you know? "90 percent of modern diseases are due to colon problems." – Dr. John Harvey Kellogg, lived to be 91*

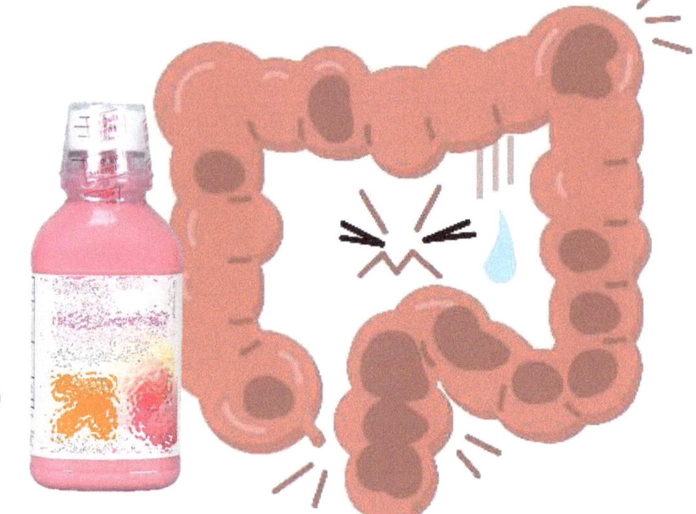

Synthetic Solutions
1.) Mange symptoms
2.) Don't address root cause
3.) Have side effects
4.) Lead to resistance build up

Natural Solutions

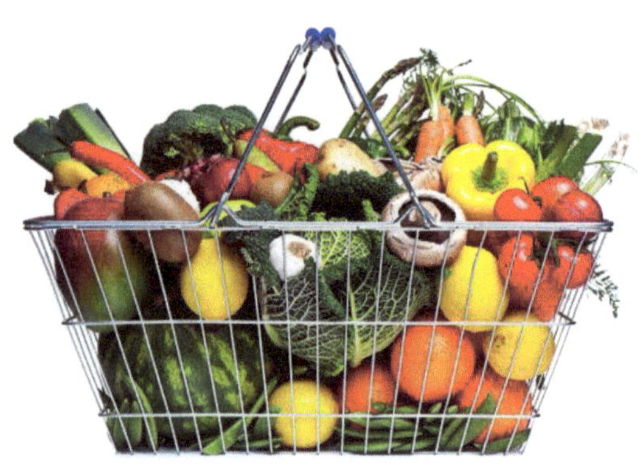

1.) **Plant based fiber**: Pushes bulk out, removes toxins, reduces plaque in arteries**
2.) **Digestive enzymes**: breaks down proteins, fats, and carbs for better absorption of nutrients
3.) **Prebiotics**: feeds probiotics to help make sure they stay alive
4.) **Probiotics**: Nourishes gut flora with good bacteria which release B Vitamins
5.) **Peppermint, ginger, fennel**

*Source: The Green Smoothies Diet, Openshaw 2007
**Source: Forks over knives, 2011

Problem #4 Low Energy

Did You Know? Processed foods destroy your *endocrine system*. Your *endocrine system* consists of hormone regulating glands that stimulate your metabolism, reproduction, blood pressure, and appetite.

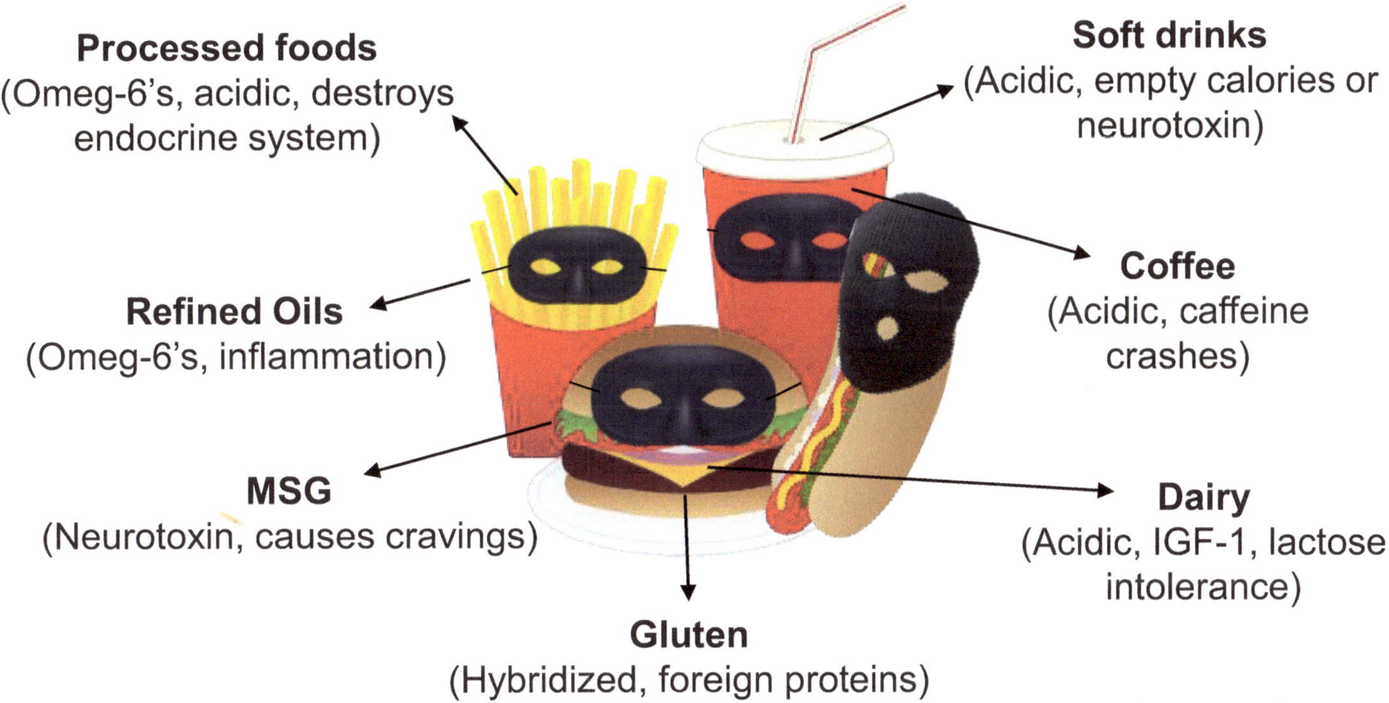

The **Standard American Diet** aka the "SAD" Crew can rob your body of what it needs the most (i.e. nutrients)

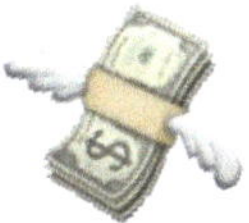 They can rob your body of vitamins, minerals, & nutrients leaving you feeling drained

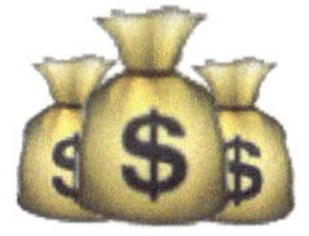 They can rob your body of enzymes needed for proper digestion and absorption of nutrients

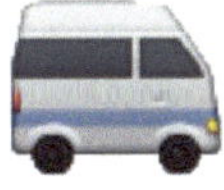 They can give you *free radicals* that do "Van-Damage" to the DNA in your cells and weaken your immune system

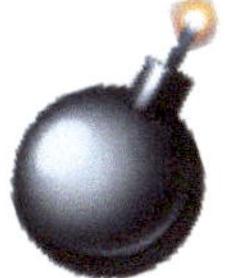 They can give you internal inflammation which leads to more pain and side effects

Problem #5: Overweight

*The statistics are stunning! 34% of Americans are obese and 32% are overweight. That means exactly 2/3 of Americans need to lose weight. Obesity has doubled since 1980**

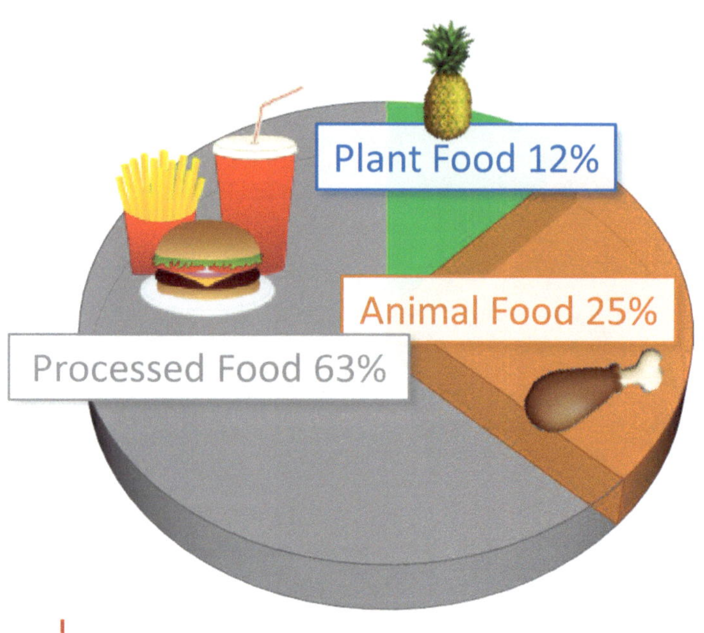

Standard American Diet (SAD)**

According to the International Agency for Research on Cancer, 80% of all cancers are attributed to environmental factors rather than genetic factors and carcinogenic chemicals and toxins can cause serious illness and disease

The 5 Headed Dragon of Chronic Western Disease (CWD)***

1. Heart disease
2. Breast Cancer
3. Prostate Cancer
4. Diabetes
5. Obesity

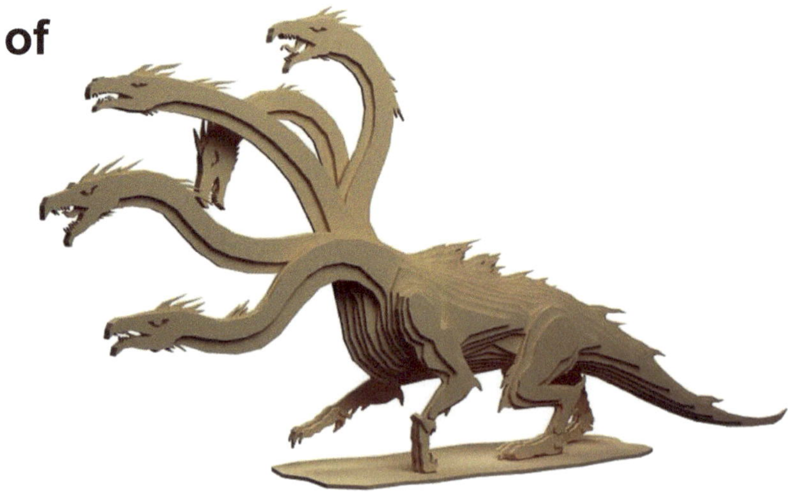

*Source: National Center for Health Statistics
**Source: USDA Economic Research Service, 2009
***Source: 12 Steps to Wholefoods, 2011; www.foodmatters.tv

Problem #5 Cont...

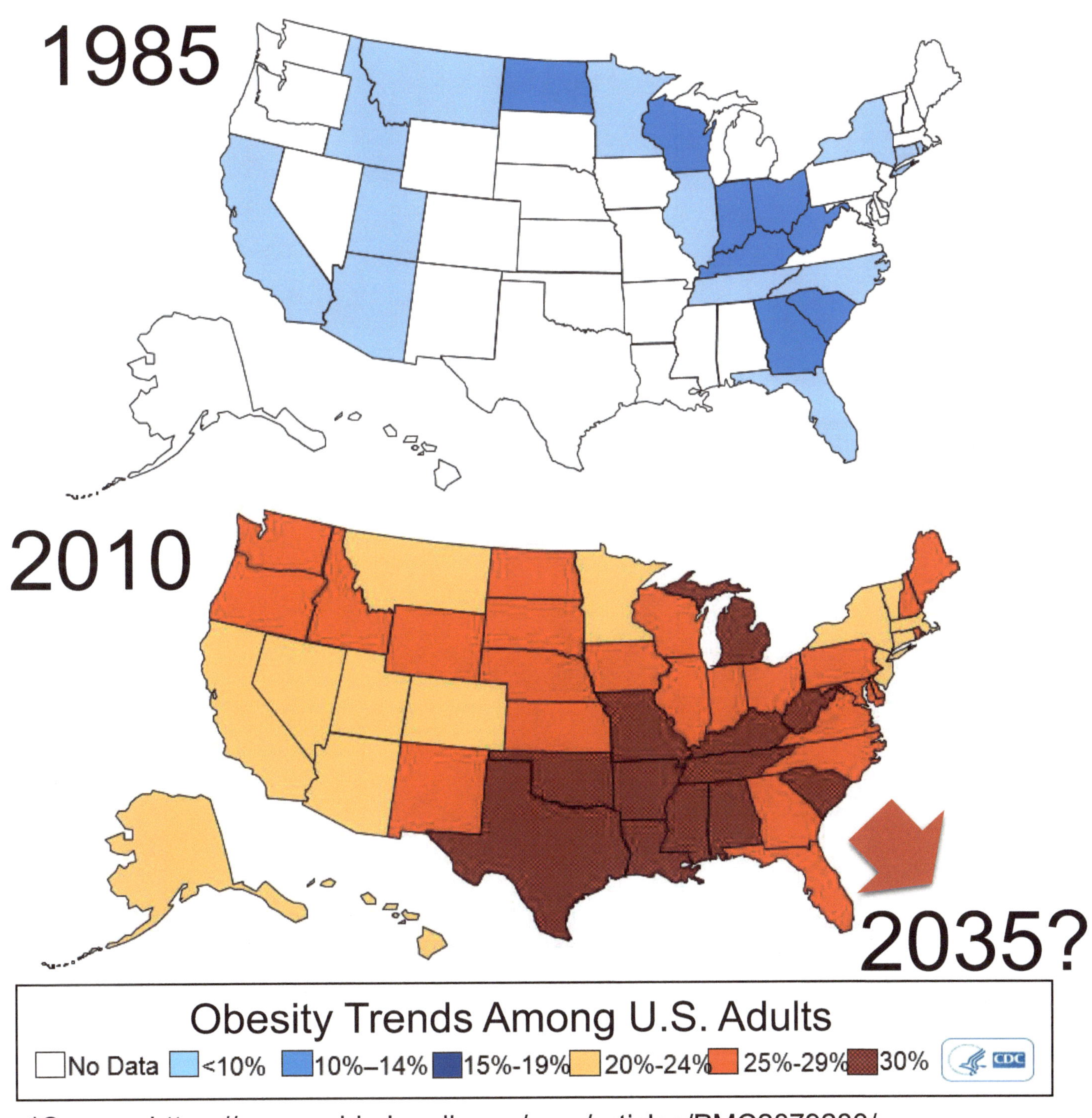

*Source: https://www.ncbi.nlm.nih.gov/pmc/articles/PMC2879283/

Problem #6: Obesity

*__Did you know?__ The __Total__ Healthcare costs in 2015 (U.S.) will equal __Just__ the cost of treating diabetes and obesity in 2035 (U.S.).**

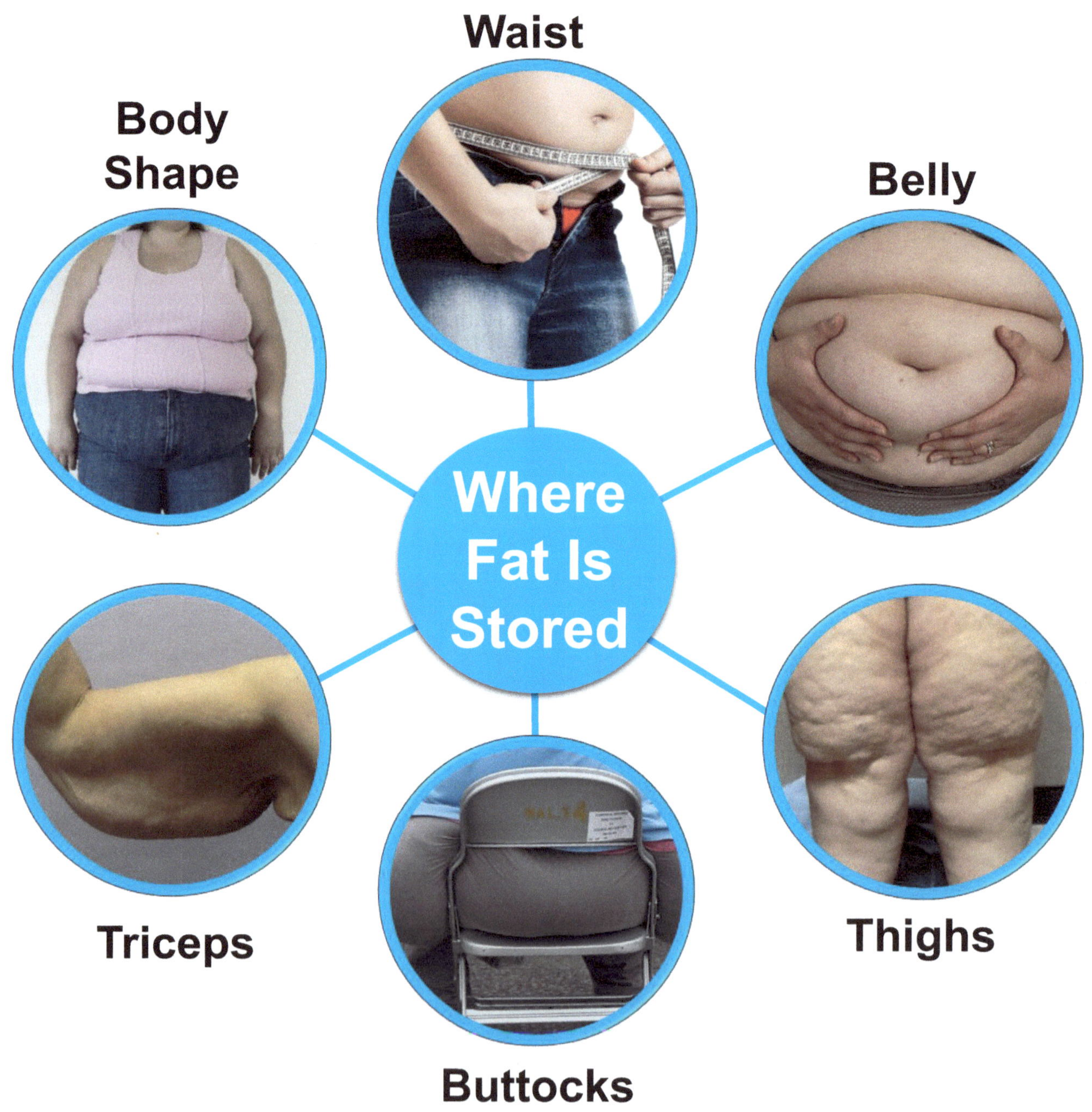

Problem #7: Healthcare Costs

Did you know? *75-90% of doctor visits are due to stress related ailments and complaints and up to 50% of Corporate profits are going to healthcare costs around diet & lifestyle. In other words, stress is going up for families.*

Direct Costs*

 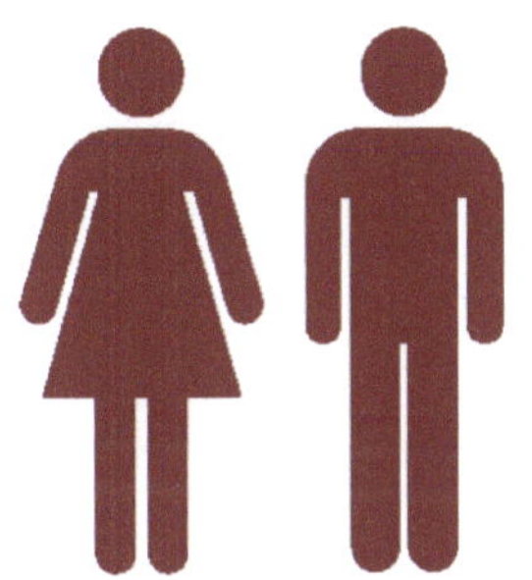 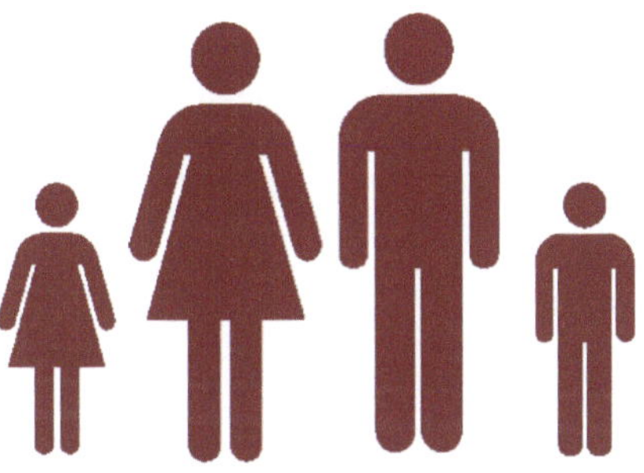

Single: $4,950

Couples or Single Parents: $9,900

Family: $17,550

Indirect Costs

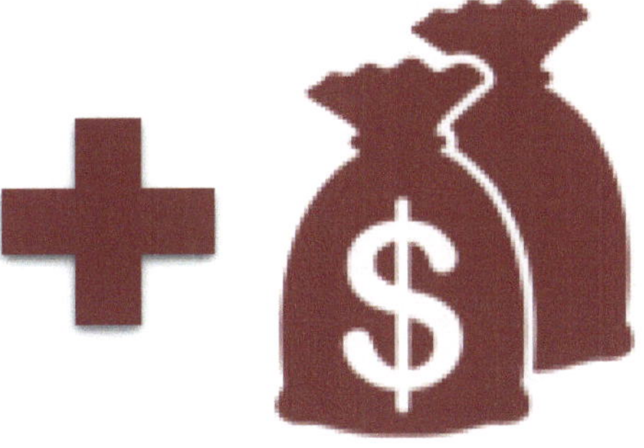

- Absenteeism
- Presenteeism
- Low Morale
- High Stress
- Low Retention
- High Turnover

The Plant Powered Solution

As growing numbers of people face health crises, the data on the protective and restorative power of a more plant-based diet becomes more compelling.

Years of food fad cycles in the Standard American Diet (aka S-A-D) have left followers suffering unnecessary health problems like cardiovascular disease, obesity, type 2 diabetes, inflammation, low energy, and the list goes on.

Growing research continues to support what many have experienced, a more **plant-based diet*** is lower in calories and dense in the nutrients that heal, protect and sustain your health, even reversing years of chronic conditions.

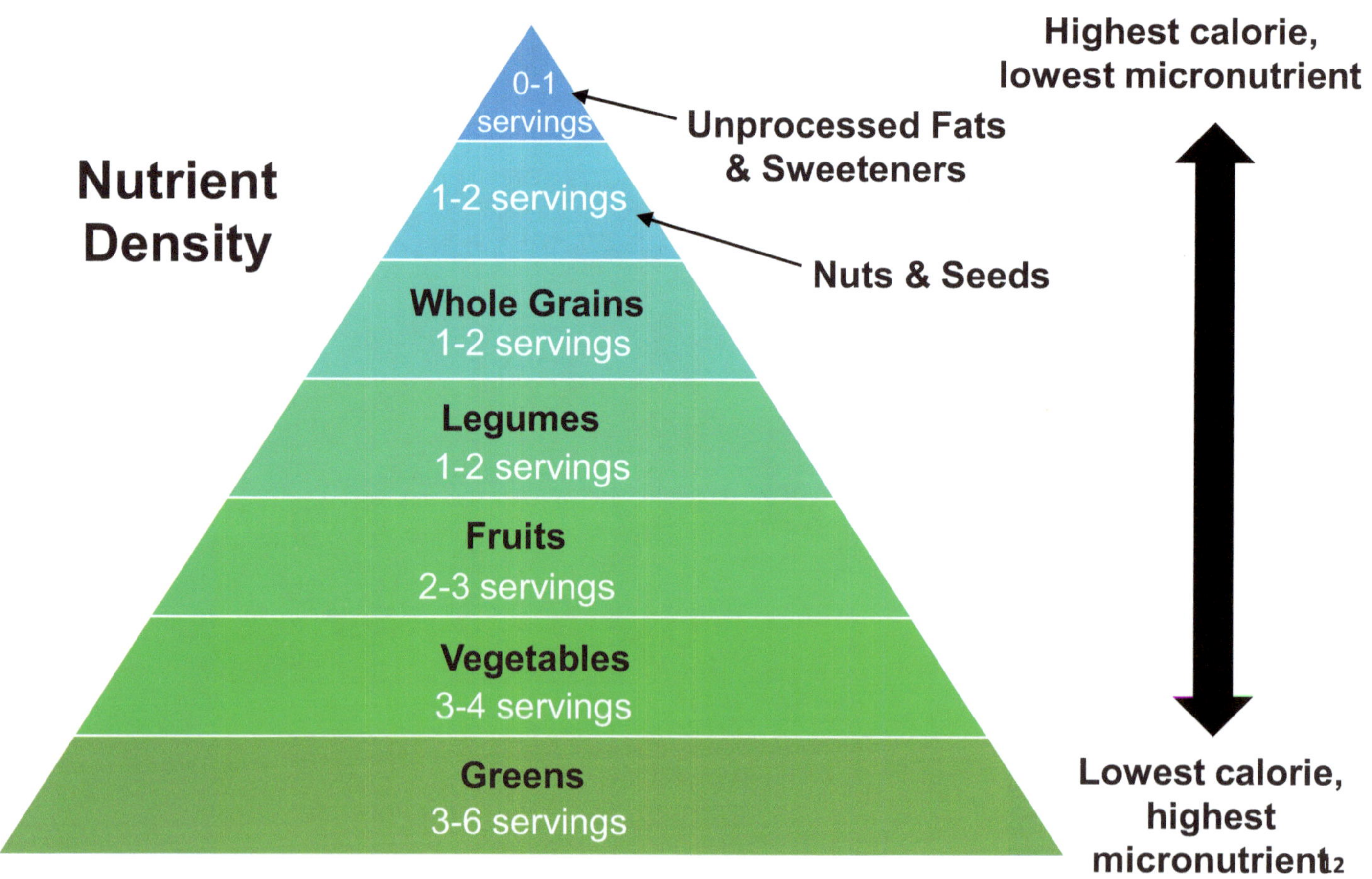

The Plant Powered Solution

Good nutrition is simple. You don't have to obsess about calories or macronutrient breakdown.

It's important to root the lifestyle in habits. Your body will rediscover it's natural craving for whole, natural foods. Better digestion, fewer cravings, increased emotional stability, weight control, and more energy are some of the many benefits of unprocessed, simple nutrition.

Oxford/Cornell China Study*

- Largest nutritional study in human history with 6500 people
- Showed that eating 95% or more plant based dramatically reduced risk of heart disease, cancer, and autoimmune diseases

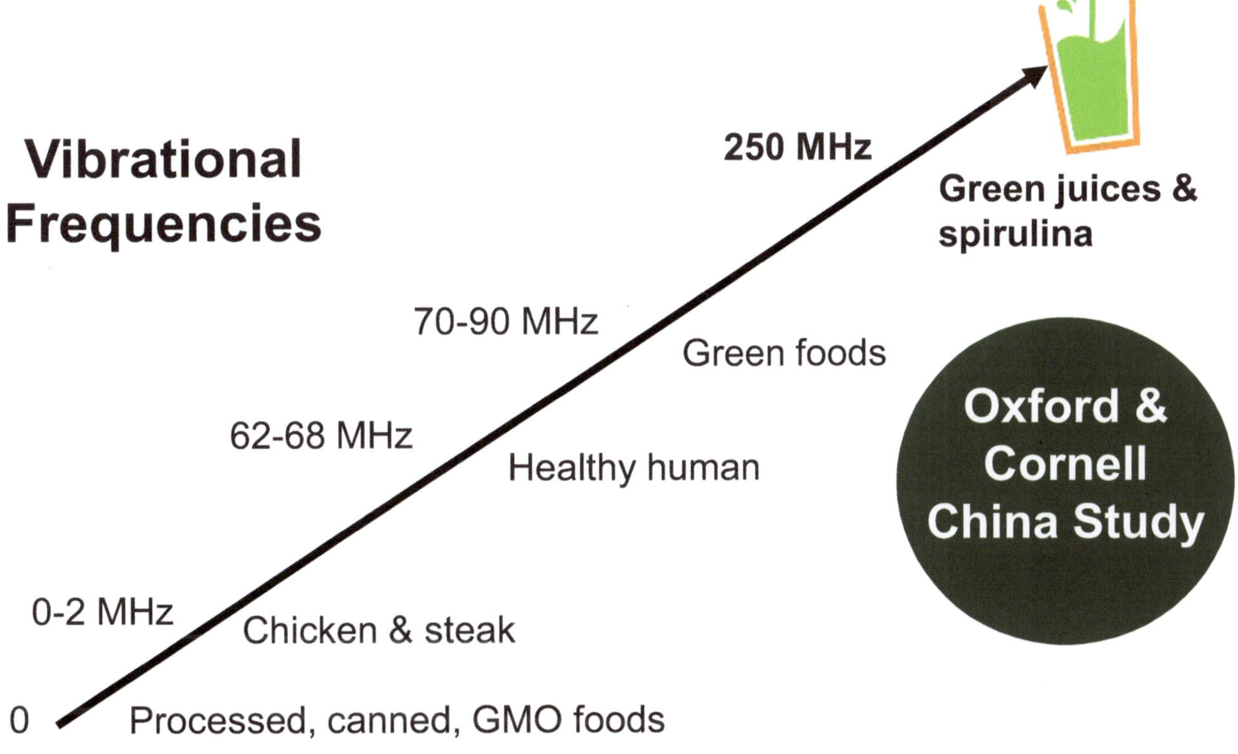

*Source: How to eat right in the real world, 2013; Drs. David Katz, MD, and Stephanie Meller, MD, Yale University, Annual Reviews, March 2014; T. Colin Campbell, PhD, The China Study, 2004.

Why Your "Why" Matters

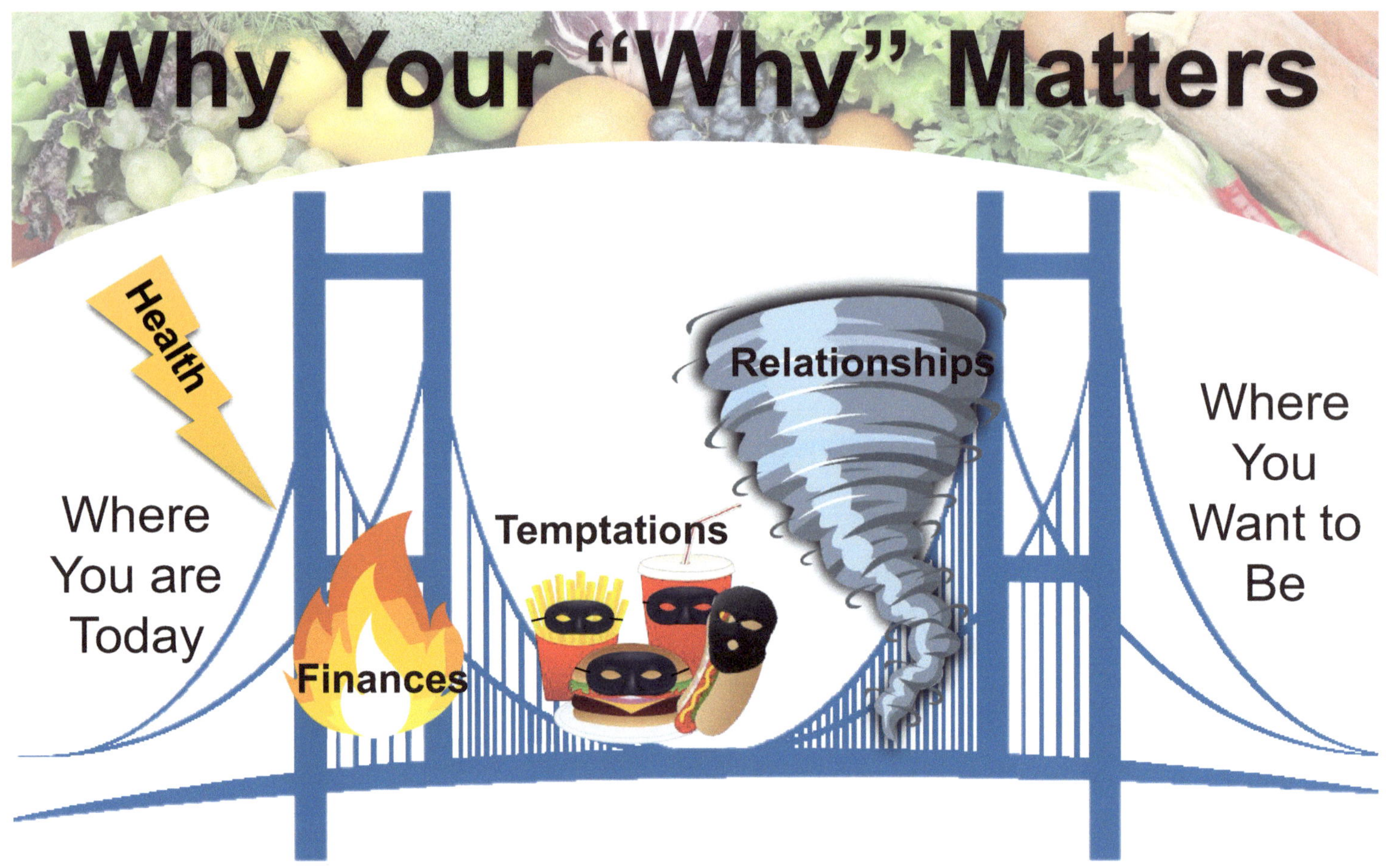

Top 3 Life Challenges That Will Test Your Why

1.) Your Health: Health concerns tend to happen just how lightning strikes, random and all of a sudden. These can include stress, low energy, digestive upset, trouble sleeping, sickness, or other health issues. The stronger you "Why," the better you can weather this storm.

2.) Your Finances: These can include living on a fixed income, living paycheck to paycheck, being on foods stamps or welfare, having a lot of debt, or being laid off. These are like a wildfire because they can destroy a lot of areas in your life in a very little amount of time. This is where a strong "Why" also comes in.

3.) Your Relationships: Conflict with a significant other, husband, wife, or family member, the passing of a loved one (without a will), or recovering from a divorce are some areas of our life that can test your why. Conflict is inevitable, but you can manage it better when you develop your skills in this area by focusing on truth and understanding (Source: How to Solve Your People Problems, Alan Godwin).

Bottom Line: The stronger your "Why," the stronger your bridge will be from getting from where you are today to where you want to be with your health and wellness goals.

BodySMITH-ing

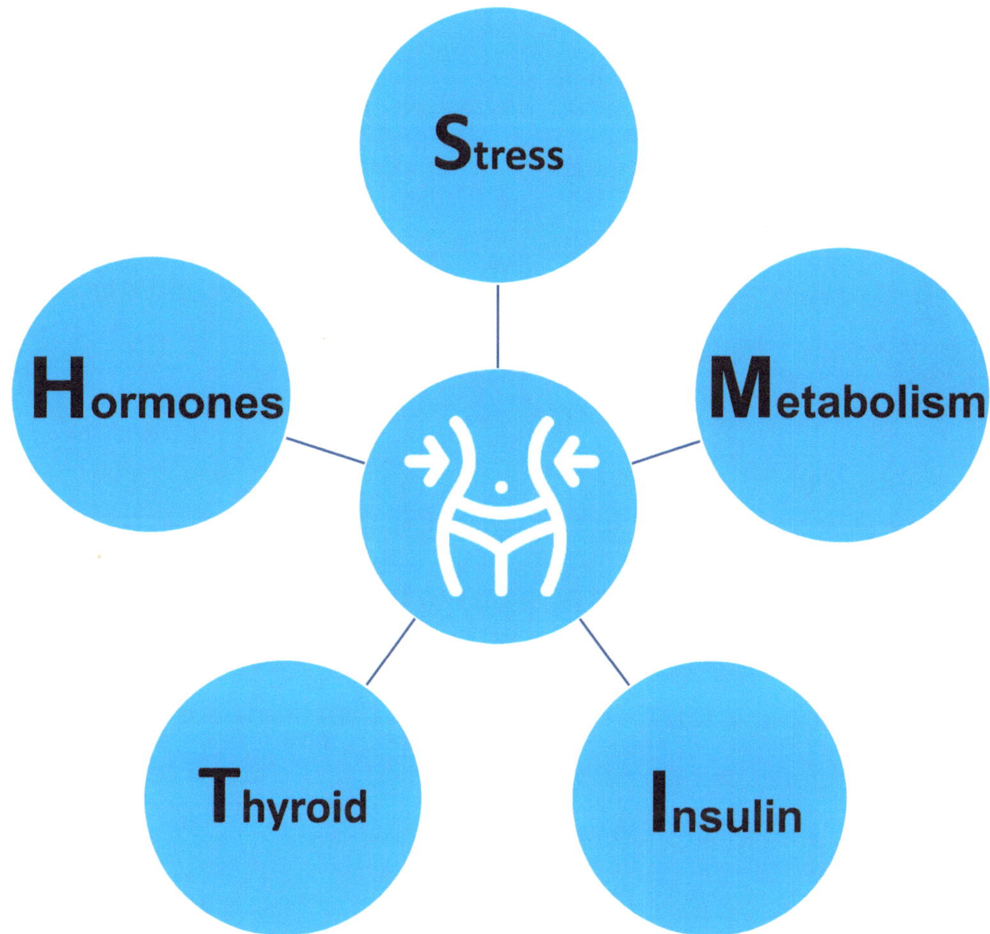

Stress
Metabolism
Insulin
Thyroid
Hormones

Eating right and exercise are the two most important factors for maintaining a healthy body weight. Other factors that influence your weight include your stress, metabolism, insulin, thyroid, and hormones. The BodySMITH-ing principle is one of the core concepts that is important to understand in addition to the FAN Rich Foods principle.

BodySMITH-ing

*A Blacksmith is a person that makes and repairs things with iron and metal by hand. Body-**SMITH**-ing is how you can reach your ideal body weight by understanding the top 5 things that affect it below.*

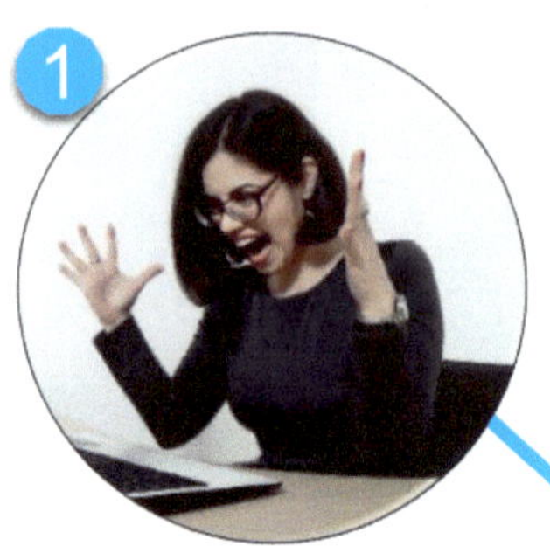

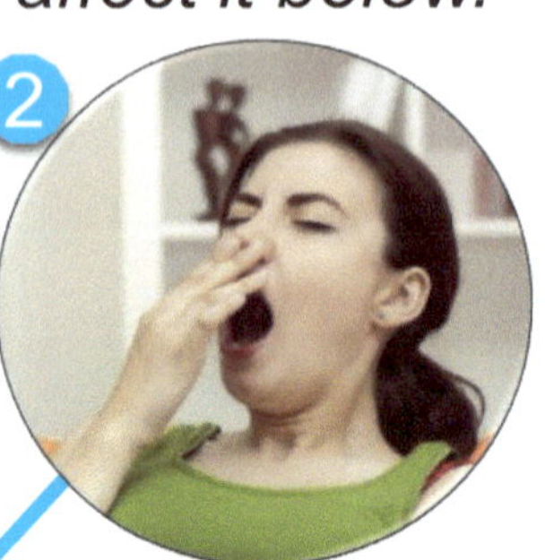

A slow **Metabolism** starts to set in after the age of 40 and is negatively affected by processed foods, which is why natural metabolism boosters are important for feeling active and young.

Stress can make you feel like you're out of control of a situation. Eating comfort foods can be just that, comforting, but excess calories not used by your body gets stored as fat.

A slow *metabolism* means that calories are being converted into energy less efficiently and any excess calories are stored as fat in your body.

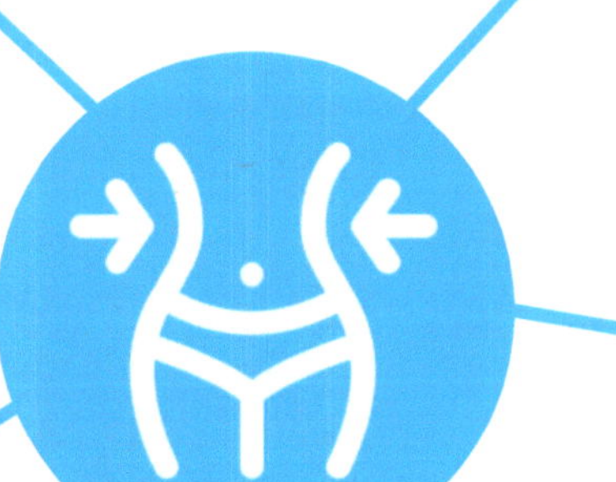

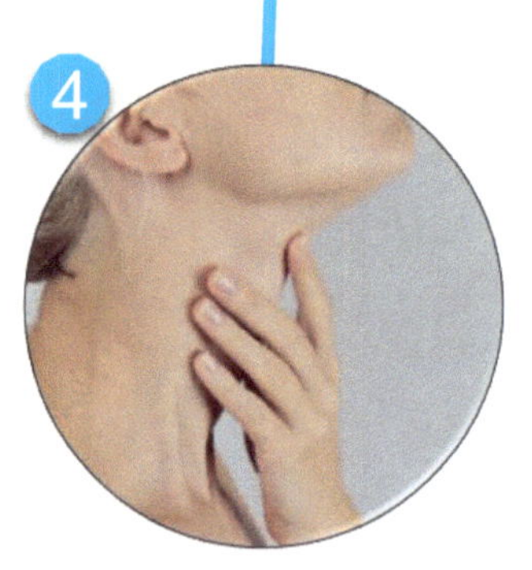

More **Insulin** in your body means that your pancreas is working harder to bring your blood sugar levels down after a meal, but your cells could be building up a resistance to the insulin over time. Excess blood sugar in your blood can lead to more sugar cravings and weight gain.

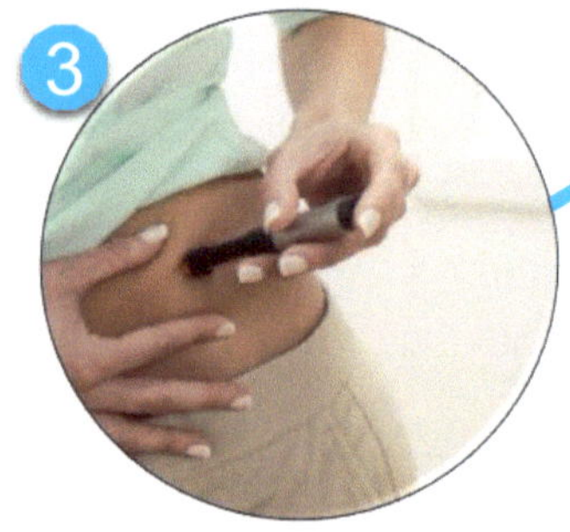

Your endocrine system uses **Hormones** to regulate metabolism, reproduction, blood pressure, appetite, and many other bodily functions. Hormone imbalance slows down your metabolism and can lead to weight gain.

When your **Thyroid** doesn't produce enough T3 and T4 hormones, then your body is not able to convert the oxygen and calories it receives into the proper amounts of energy. This decreases your metabolism and can lead to weight gain.

FAN Rich Foods

The Problem: Americans only get about 11-14 grams of fiber per day. *Cholesterol* is only found in animal foods such as meat, dairy, eggs, fish, and seafood. An imbalance of "bad" *cholesterol* can clog up your arteries with plaque and cause complications in the future.

Eating more whole foods from plant sources contributes to a *better well being*

The Solution: Fiber is only found in plant foods and getting 40+ grams of fiber per day is ideal for lowering bad or LDL cholesterol, stabilizing blood sugar, along with removing toxins with an insoluble form of fiber

The Problem: The Standard American Diet (SAD) of processed foods are nutrient void, high in inflammation causing compounds, and destroy your endocrine system.
The Solution: Leafy greens are the most nutrient dense and lowest calorie foods on the planet. These include spinach, swiss chard, kale, and collard greens.

The Problem: Free radicals get out of control from too much exposure to radiation, cigarette smoke, fried foods, processed foods, and air pollution and can damage your DNA, tissues, organs, cause cell death, and can lead to inflammation, pain, and diseases.
The Solution: The Food Antioxidant Capacity (FAC) of pomegranates is 3,309, blueberries are 2,400, and kale is 1,770. Getting more antioxidants helps to minimize and reverse free radical damage.

FAN Rich Food List

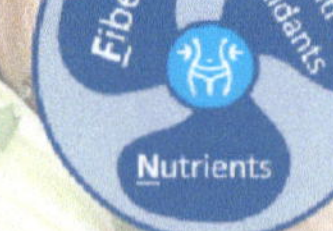

| <u>F</u>iber Rich | <u>A</u>ntioxidant Rich | <u>N</u>utrient Rich |

(Baby) Spinach
(1/3 cup, 85g)
Protein: 2g
Fiber: 3g
Calories: 20
Vitamin A: 120%
Vitamin C: 30%

(Baby) Kale Yeah!
(1 ½ cups, 84g)
Protein: 2g
Fiber: 2g
Calories: 30
Vitamin A: 100%
Vitamin C: 50%

(Baby) Chard
(1 cup, 89g)
Protein: 2g
Fiber: 2g
Calories: 20
Vitamin A: 100%
Vitamin C: 25%

(Baby) Collard Greens
(1/2 cup, 118g)
Protein: 2g
Fiber: 2g
Calories: 35
Vitamin A: 100%
Vitamin C: 20%

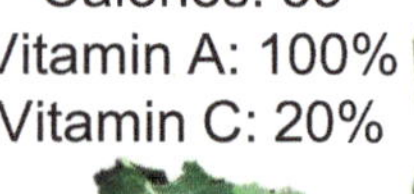
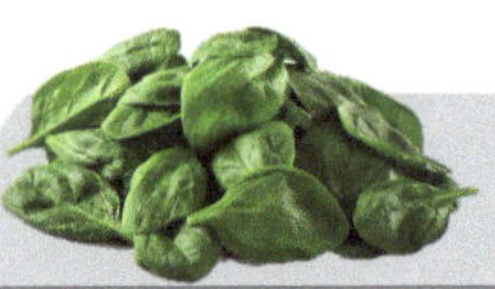
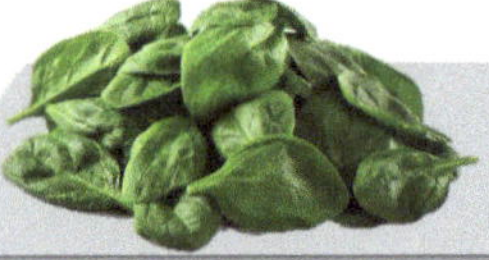

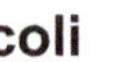

Broccoli
(7 florets, 85g)
Protein: 1g
Fiber: 2g
Calories: 30
Vitamin A: 6%
Vitamin C: 50%

Cauliflower
(1 cup, 85g)
Protein: 1g
Fiber: 1g
Calories: 25
Vitamin A: 0%
Vitamin C: 35%

White Onions
(1 cup, 160g)
Protein: 2g
Fiber: 3g
Calories: 64
Vitamin A: 0%
Vitamin C: 20%

Green Lentils
(1/4 cup, 50g)
Protein: 13g
Fiber: 15g
Calories: 180
Vitamin A: 0%
Vitamin C: 4%

Millet
(1 cup, 174g)
Protein: 6g
Fiber: 2g
Calories: 207
Vitamin A: 0%
Vitamin C: 0%

Quinoa
(1 cup, 185g)
Protein: 8g
Fiber: 5g
Calories: 222
Vitamin A: 0%
Vitamin C: 0%

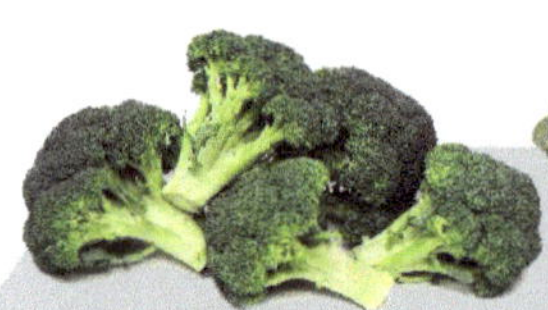
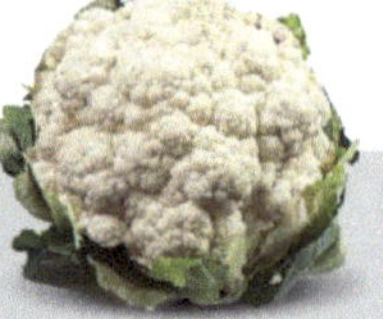
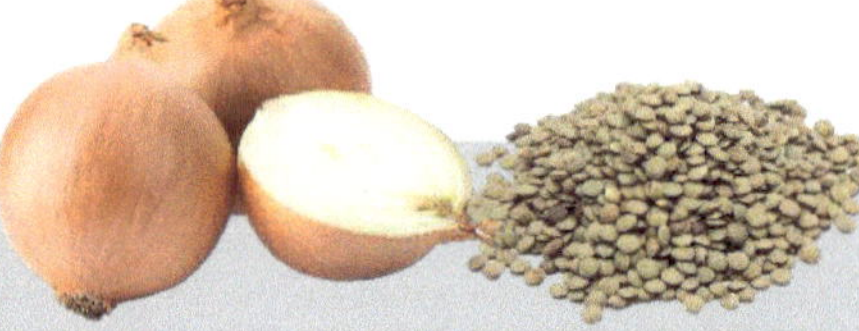
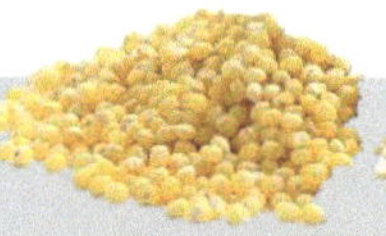
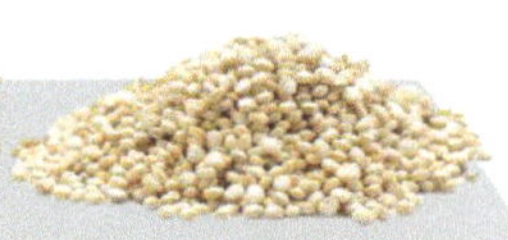

Blackberries
(1 cup, 140g)
Protein: 1g
Fiber: 7g
Calories: 80
Sugar: 15g

Blueberries
(1 cup, 140g)
Protein: 1g
Fiber: 4g
Calories: 70
Sugar: 12g

Raspberries
(1 ¼ cup, 140g)
Protein: 1g
Fiber: 2g
Calories: 60
Sugar: 6g

Strawberries
(8 of 'em, 147g)
Protein: 1g
Fiber: 2g
Calories: 50
Sugar: 6g

Mixed Berries
(1 cup, 100g)
Protein: <1g
Fiber: 2g
Calories: 50
Sugar: 7g

Apple
(Whole, 242g)
Protein: 1g
Fiber: 5g
Calories: 130
Sugar: 25g

Cherries
(3/4 cup, 140g)
Protein: 1g
Fiber: 3g
Calories: 110
Sugar: 20g

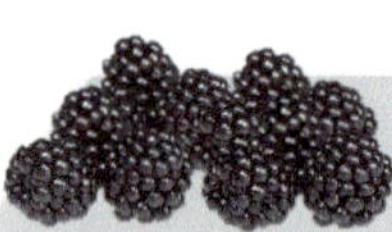
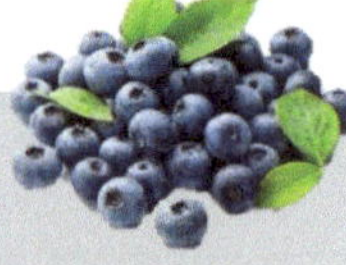
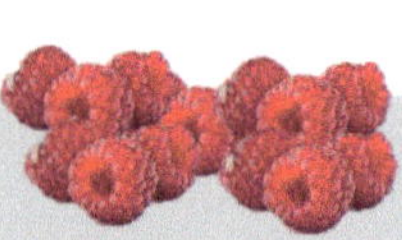
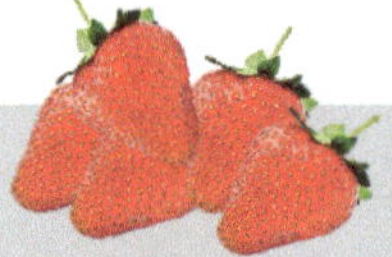
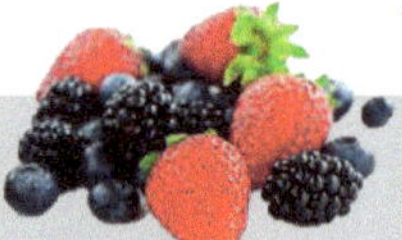
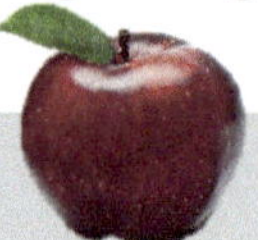
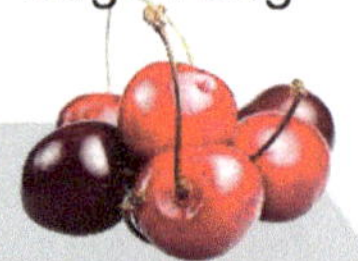

Mango
(Whole, 207g)
Protein: 1g
Fiber: 3g
Calories: 90
Sugar: 21g

Banana
(Whole, 126g)
Protein: 1g
Fiber: 3g
Calories: 110
Sugar: 19g

Peach
(Whole, 147g)
Protein: 1g
Fiber: 2g
Calories: 60
Sugar: 13g

Pineapple
(2 slices, 112g)
Protein: 1g
Fiber: 1g
Calories: 50
Sugar: 10g

Orange
(Whole, 154g)
Protein: 1g
Fiber: 3g
Calories: 80
Sugar: 14g

Lemon
(Whole, 58g)
Protein: 0g
Fiber: 2g
Calories: 15
Sugar: 2g

Lime
(Whole, 67g)
Protein: 0g
Fiber: 2g
Calories: 20
Sugar: 0g

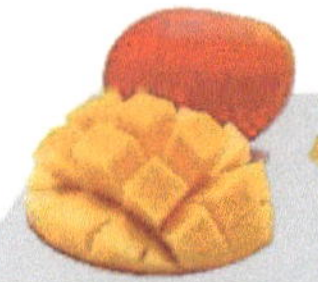
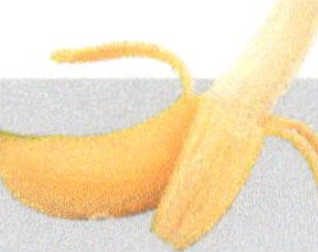
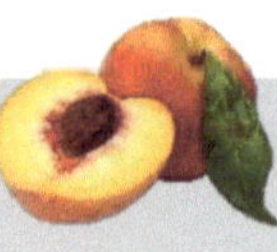
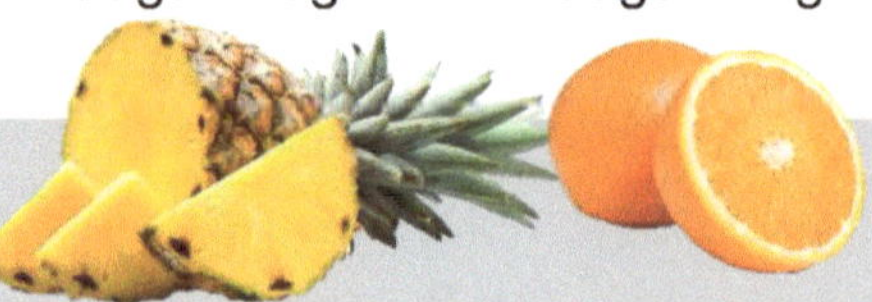
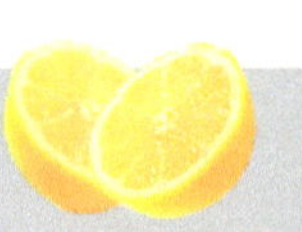
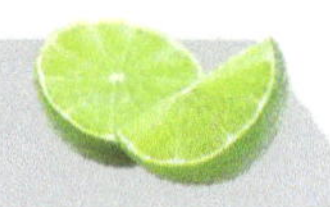

30 Day Green Smoothie Challenge*

Fiber Rich | Antioxidant Rich | Nutrient Rich

Top 3 Benefits
1.) More energy
2.) Better digestion
3.) Weight loss

*1 quart of green smoothie per day for 30 days, while eating what you normally eat and trying to minimize processed foods/fast foods.

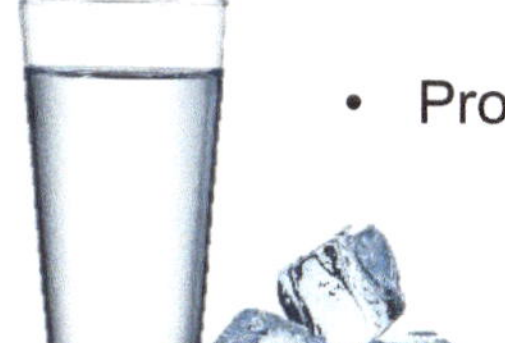

1 ½ cups alkaline or distilled water and ice
- Provides pure, refreshing, and cool experience

High Powered Blender
- Liquefies whole foods into water-like consistency for easier drinking
- Breaks down plant cell walls for better absorption

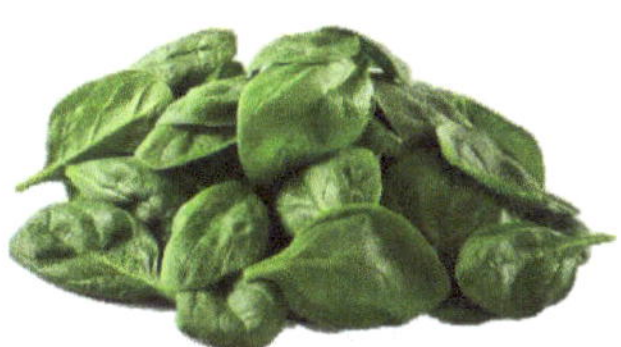

3 cups organic baby spinach
- Provides nutrient density, fiber, enzymes, and protein

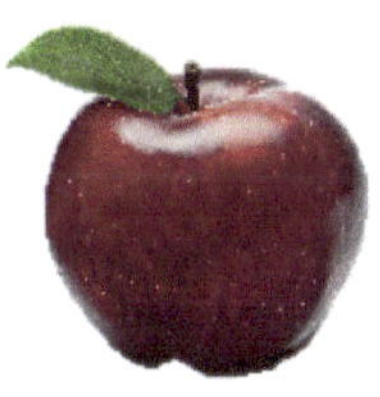

1 organic apple
- Provides fiber, flavor, and enzymes

1 organic banana
- Provides flavor, creaminess, & enzymes

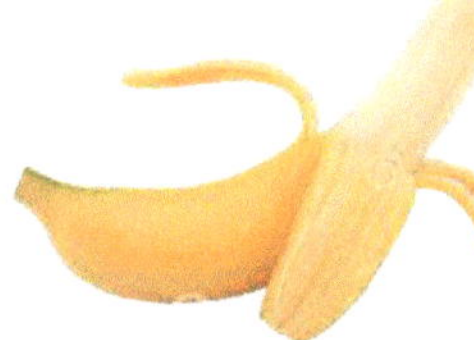

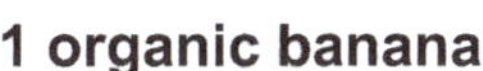
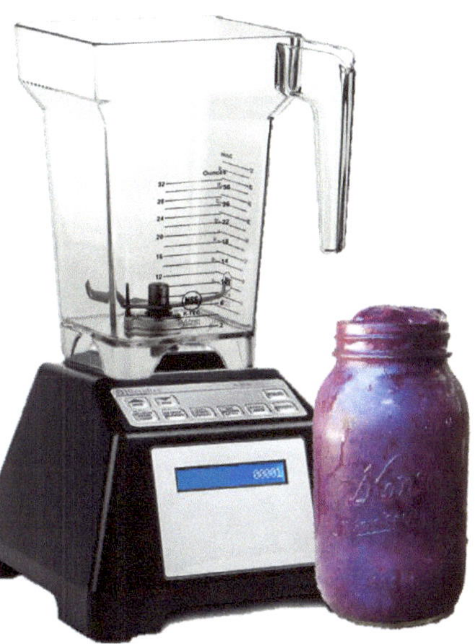

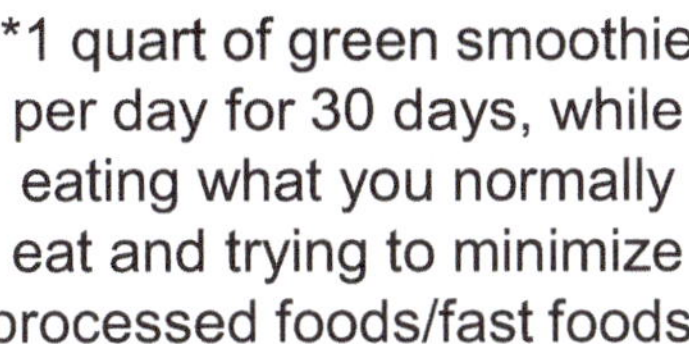

2 medium organic swiss chard leaves
- Provides nutrient density, fiber, enzymes, & protein

Did You Know?
Fiber is only found in **plant foods**. *Fiber* helps lower "bad" cholesterol, stabilize blood sugar, and remove harmful toxins from your body. Eating more whole foods from plant sources contributes to a *better well being*.

2 cups frozen organic mixed berries
- Provides nutrients, fiber, and flavor

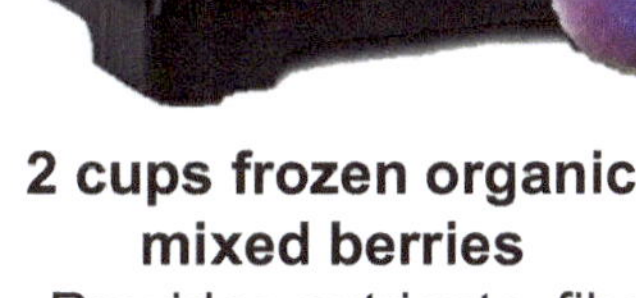

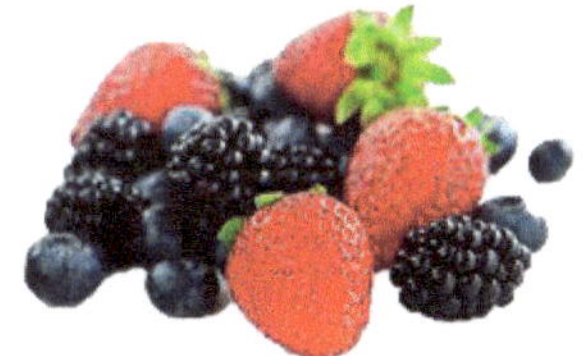

1 scoop organic plant based protein powder (Orgain)
- Helps build lean muscle, burn fat, provide more fullness, and balance blood sugar

Directions: In a high powered blender, combine water, ice, and greens and blend for 30 seconds until smooth. Add fruit, protein powder, and blend for another 30 seconds until smooth. Makes about 1 quart (32 ounces) and keeps for 48 hours in the fridge.

Traffic Light Take A Bite

Eat

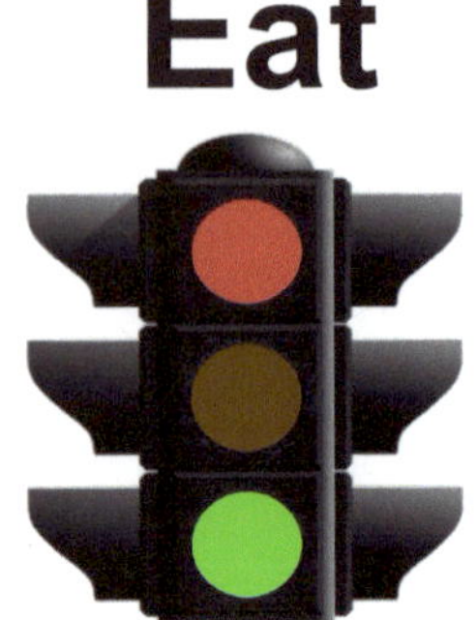

Fact: Greens are the most nutrient dense and lowest calorie food on the planet*

Greens
3-6 servings

Vegetables
3-4 servings

Fruits
2-3 servings

Legumes
1-2 servings

Whole Grains
1-2 servings

Nuts & Seeds → 1-2 servings

- Chard, bok choy, collard greens, spinach, kale

- Carrots, sweet potatoes, beets, celery, bell peppers, green beans, onions, cucumbers, broccoli

- Apples, bananas, oranges, pears, mango, pineapple, watermelon, cantaloupe, berries, avocados

- Lentils, hummus, black beans, pinto beans, kidney beans, navy beans, white beans, lima beans

- Millet, quinoa, wild rice, black rice, brown rice

- Raw and unsalted: almonds, cashews, pecans, brazil nuts, sunflower seeds, pumpkins seeds

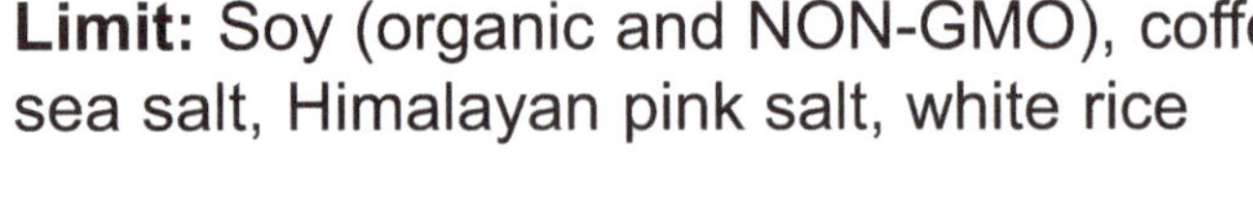

Unprocessed Fats & Sweeteners → 0-1 servings

Limit: Soy (organic and NON-GMO), coffee, sea salt, Himalayan pink salt, white rice

- Olive oil, avocado oil, coconut oil, sesame oil, raw agave, coconut sugar, maple syrup, raw honey, stevia

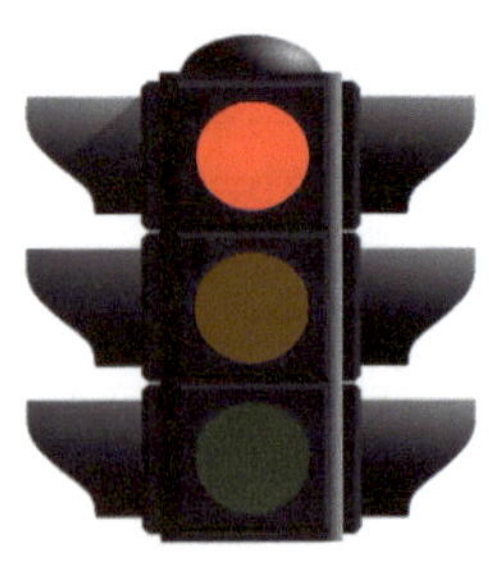

Avoid: Organic & free range meat (beef, chicken, eggs), wild caught seafood, processed foods (frozen or TV dinners, hamburgers, hot dogs, pizza), fried foods (french fries, fried chicken, chips), alcohol (beer, liquor, wine, whiskey), caffeinated sodas, diet sodas, energy drinks, sports drinks, tobacco, pork, dairy (milk, cheese, yogurt, ice cream), wheat (white bread, wheat bread, white pasta), iodized salt, white sugar, Splenda, aspartame, sucralose, (high fructose) corn syrup, food dyes, artificial flavorings, MSG, refined oils (canola, corn, soy, vegetable)

***Sources:** Joel Fuhrman, MD; Douglas Graham, DC; Neal A. Barnard, MD; T. Colin Campbell, PhD; Caldwell Esselstyn, MD

Fill Up Before You Calorie Up

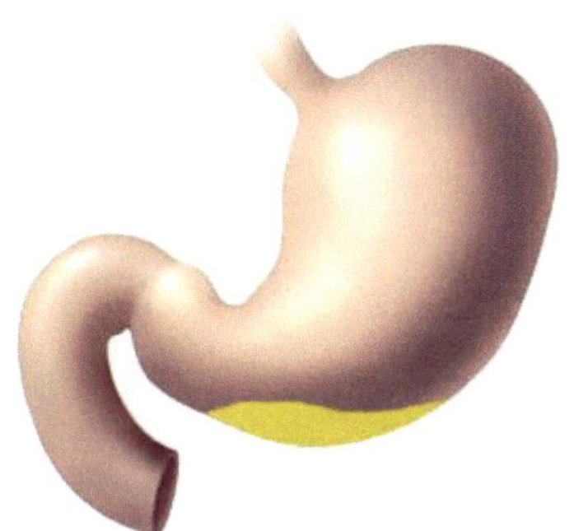

400 Calories of **Oil**

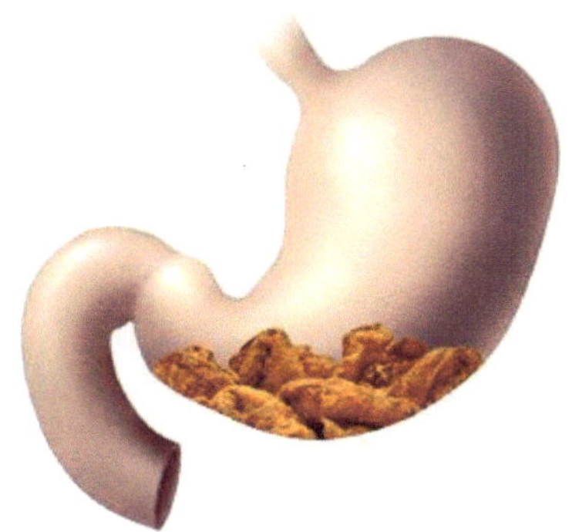

400 Calories of **Chicken**

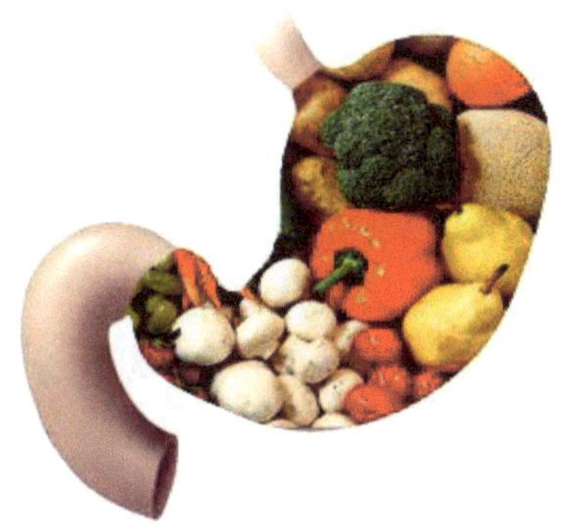

400 Calories of **Vegetables**

Nutrient dense foods are low in calorie, fill you up quite well, and are a great source of lean protein, fiber, and healthy fats. Your stomach has stretch receptors that can tell how full it is, and it's good to know that eating more whole foods that are raw and organic solves the problem of counting calories. Count on nutrition filling you up!

Superfoods 101

What Are Superfoods?

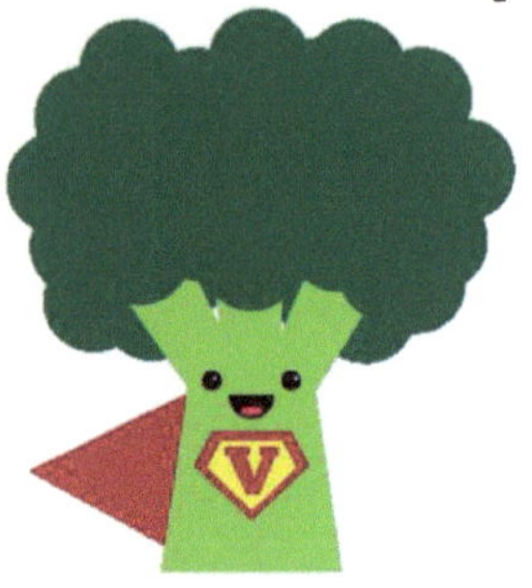

Superfoods are nutrient-dense, natural compounds that come with many proven health benefits. They are good sources of vitamins, minerals, omega-3 fatty acids, probiotics, or antioxidants!

Delicious Superfood Shake Recipe

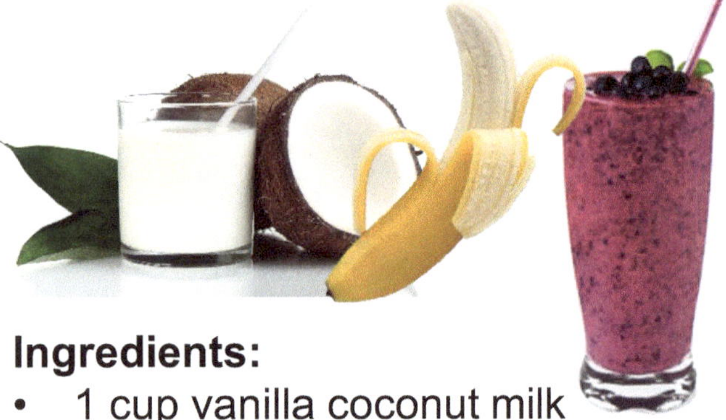

Ingredients:
- 1 cup vanilla coconut milk
- 1/2 cup frozen organic blueberries
- 1 ripe banana (peeled)
- 1 scoop plant based protein powder
- 1 tablespoon chia seeds or flax meal
- 1 scoop green superfood powder

Directions:
Add all the ingredients to a high powered blender and blend for 30 seconds or until smooth.

Top 10 Superfoods

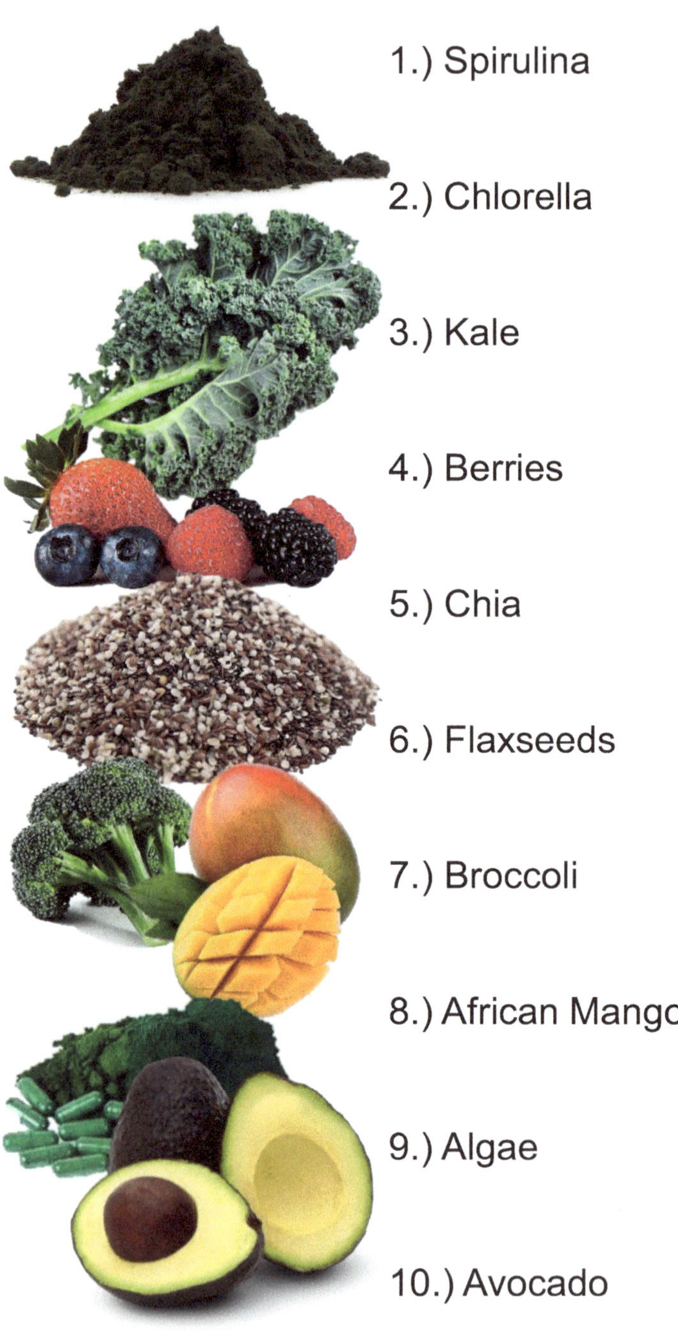

1.) Spirulina

2.) Chlorella

3.) Kale

4.) Berries

5.) Chia

6.) Flaxseeds

7.) Broccoli

8.) African Mango

9.) Algae

10.) Avocado

Note: Anything "Green" above will not taste good by itself, possibly give off a weird smell, and should be used according to one of my recipes to avoid a bad experience. They still have Superfood Powers so don't give up on them! ;-)

Taste The Rainbow

Tip: Eat fruits & veggies in front of your kids or grandkids & lead by example since research suggests a child needs 20+ exposures before accepting it.

Why Taste The Rainbow

- **Did you know?** 38% of adolescents and 36% of adults report consuming fruit less than one time daily.*
- **The Problem:** Advertising has told us what to eat instead of why to eat it so french fries, ketchup, and juice is how most people get their serving.

Why All Colors Matter

Phytochemicals are plant chemicals that only certain colors of plants produce and have specific benefits like anti-aging, energy, stamina, and protecting cells from free radical damage.

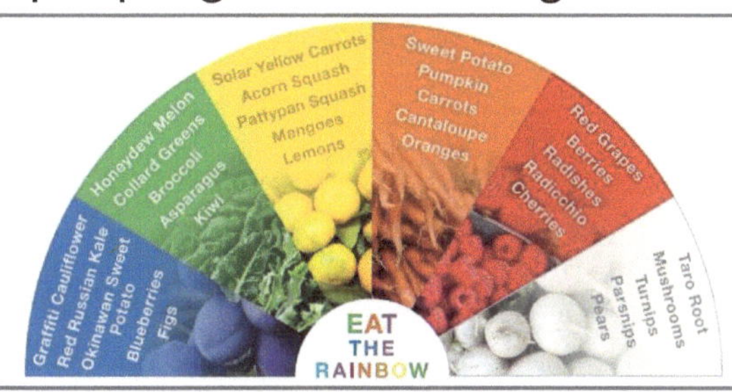

Taste The Rainbow

Tip #2: Next time you're at the grocery store, remember to buy "ROY G BIV" (i.e. Red, Orange, Yellow, Green, Blue, Indigo, & Violet) whole foods.

COLOR	PHYTOCHEMICAL		FRUITS & VEGGIES
1.) Red	Lycopene		Tomatoes, tomato products, juices, soups, sauces
2.) Red-Purple	Anthocyanins & polyphenols		Blackberries, raspberries, grapes, blueberries, eggplant, red cabbage
3.) Orange	Alpha & Beta carotene		Carrots, mangos, pumpkins
4.) Orange-Yellow	Beta Cryptozanthin & flavonoids		Cantaloupe, peaches, papaya, tangerines, oranges, pineapples
5.) Yellow-Green	Lutein & Zeaxanthin		Avocado, honeydew, pears, apples
6.) Green	Glucosinolates & indoles		Spinach, broccoli, bok choi, kale, collards, chard
7.) White-Green	Allyl sulfides		Leeks, garlic, onion, chives

*Source: State Indicator Report on Fruits and Vegetables (2013), published by CDC
**Disclaimer: These statements have not been evaluated by the FDA and are not intended to diagnose, treat or cure any disease. Results may vary depending on starting point, goals and effort.

Whole Food Recipes

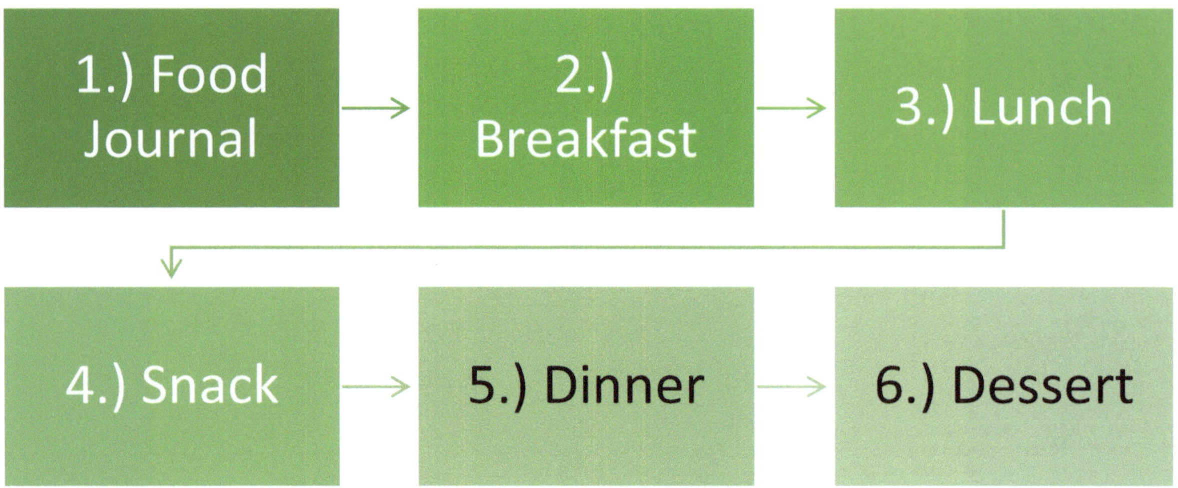

The goal of these Delicious Whole Foods Recipes is to help make wellness a lifestyle in addition to the supplements you'll be using. The first and most important thing you can do to improve your health is to eat right.

This means eating more live and whole foods and minimizing or eliminating processed foods, which will improve the effectiveness of your supplements and essential oils.

The next step is to not focus on diets or fads, but document everything that you eat in a food journal for one week. That includes what you eat for breakfast, lunch, snacks, dinner, and dessert and slowly start to replace overly processed ingredients with more whole food, high fiber, high antioxidant, and high nutrient density alternatives.

Choosing organic and non-GMO verified foods is also a another best practice. I included some recipes to start off with in conjunction to the 30 Day Green Smoothie Challenge and is just the tip of the iceberg of what you can get with a more plant based lifestyle.

Green Smoothie

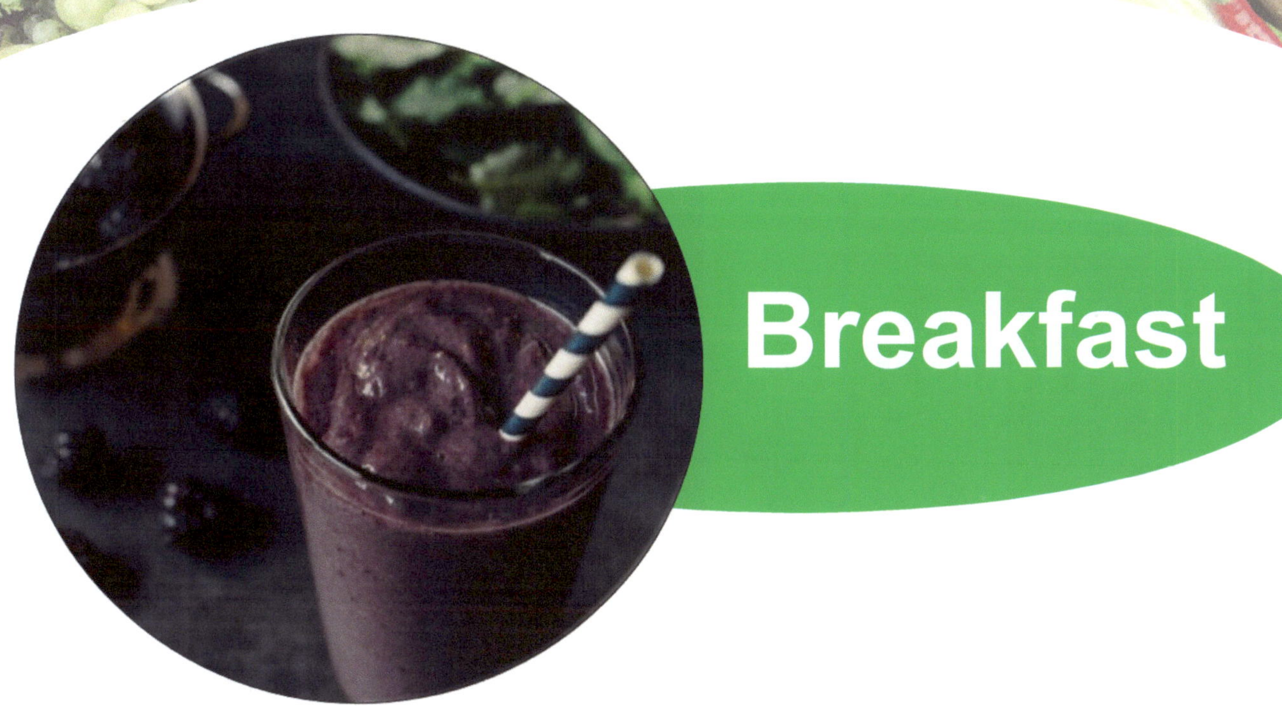

Breakfast

Ingredients:

- 1 ½ cup distilled or alkaline water
- 1 cup ice
- 2 large leaves of organic chard
- 3 handfuls of organic spinach
- 2 cups frozen organic mixed berries (12 oz bag)
- 1 banana (peeled)
- 1 scoop plant based protein powder (Orgain)
- ½ scoop sprouted flax (optional)

Directions:

In a high-speed blender, blend water, ice, and greens for 30 seconds. Add berries, banana, protein powder, flax, and blend until smooth.

Chocoholic Smoothie

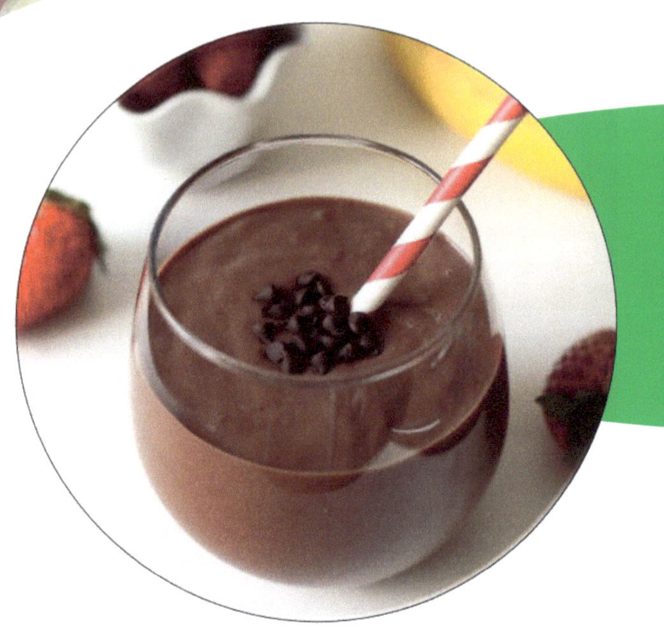

Breakfast

Bonus:
Add (vegan) chocolate chips on top for a flavorful boost

Ingredients:

- 1 ½ cups chocolate almond milk
- ½ cup ice
- 1 ½ cups organic (baby) kale
- 1 banana
- ½ cup organic strawberries
- 1 scoop plant based protein powder (Orgain)

Directions:

- In a high-speed blender, blend almond milk, ice, and baby kale for 30 seconds. Add banana, strawberries, agave, and plant based protein powder and blend until smooth.

Beginner Green Smoothie

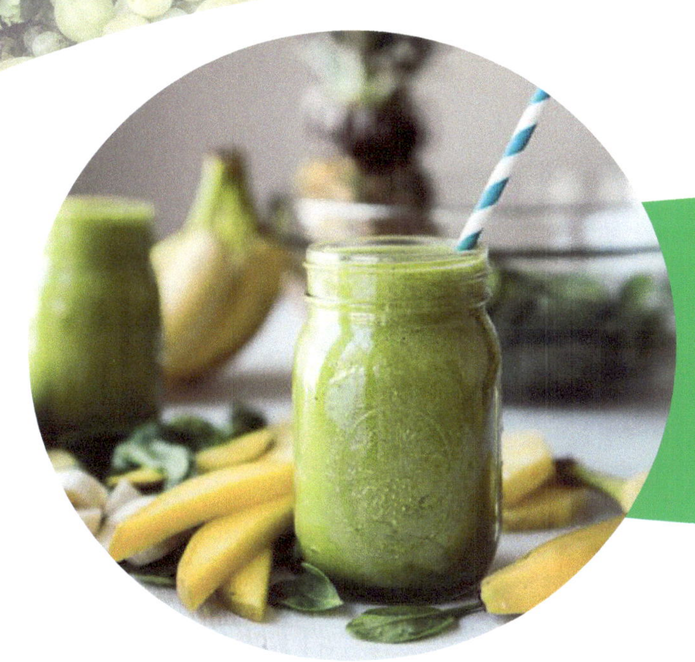

Breakfast

Ingredients:

- 2 cup water
- 1 cup ice
- 3 handfuls of organic spinach
- 2 large leaves of chard
- 1 apple (cored/seeded)
- 1 banana (peeled)
- 1 orange (peeled)
- 1 scoop plant based protein powder (Orgain)

Directions:

- In a high-speed blender, blend water, ice, and greens for 30 seconds. Add apple, banana, orange, plant based protein powder, and blend until smooth.

Split Pea Soup

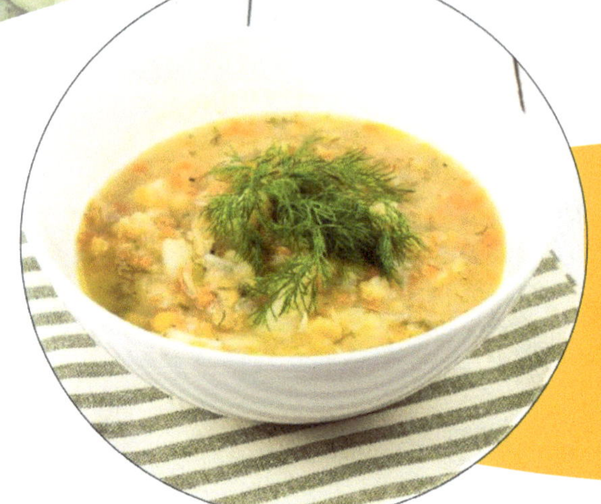

Lunch

Ingredients:

- 1 ½ tsp extra virgin olive oil
- 1 yellow onion, chopped
- 1 bay leaf
- 1 ½ cloves garlic, minced
- 1 cup dried split peas, rinsed well
- ½ cup brown rice, rinsed well
- 7 cups water
- 2 carrots, chopped
- 2 stalks celery, chopped
- 1 ½ potatoes, diced
- 2 Tbsp. dried (or 4 Tbsp. fresh) parsley
- 1 ½ tsp. dried basil
- 1 ½ tsp. dried thyme
- 1/3 tsp. freshly ground black pepper
- 1 Tbsp. sea salt

Directions:

1.) In a large pot over medium-high heat, sauté the onion and garlic in the oil until the onions are semi-clear in color

2.) Add the peas, rice, bay leaves, salt, and water

3.) Bring to a boil and reduce heat to low

4.) Simmer for 20 min., stirring occasionally

5.) Add the carrots, celery, potatoes, parsley, basil, thyme, and pepper

6.) Simmer for 30 min. until the vegetables are tender

Hearty Vegetarian Chili

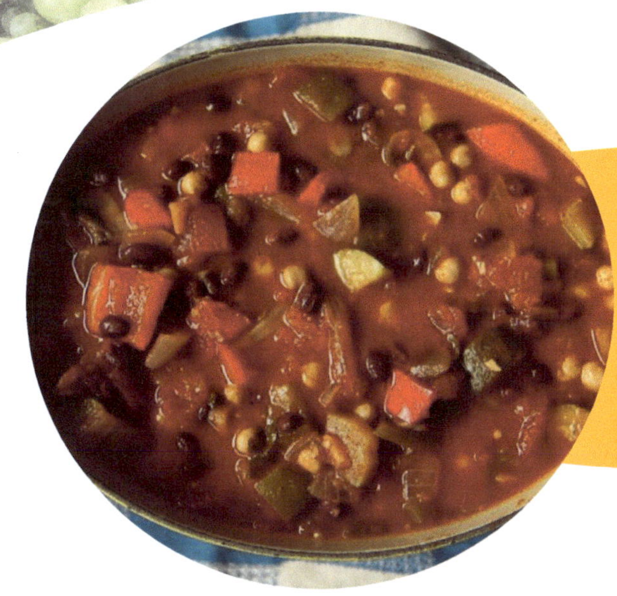

Ingredients:

- 2 cups dried pinto beans (soaked for 8 hours)
- 6 cups water
- 1 diced yellow onion
- 1 diced bell pepper (red, yellow, or green)
- 2 cans organic tomato paste
- 2 (14 ½ oz) cans organic diced tomatoes with juice
- 1 tablespoon chili powder
- 1 tablespoon garlic powder
- ¼ teaspoon sea salt
- ½ teaspoon black pepper
- 1-2 bay leaves

Directions:

- In a very large stock pot, bring the 6 cups of water with the soaked beans to a boil then simmer for 1-2 hours until they are almost tender. Add all the remaining ingredients and simmer for 1 hour then serve. Serves 8-10 people

Garden Salad With Dressing

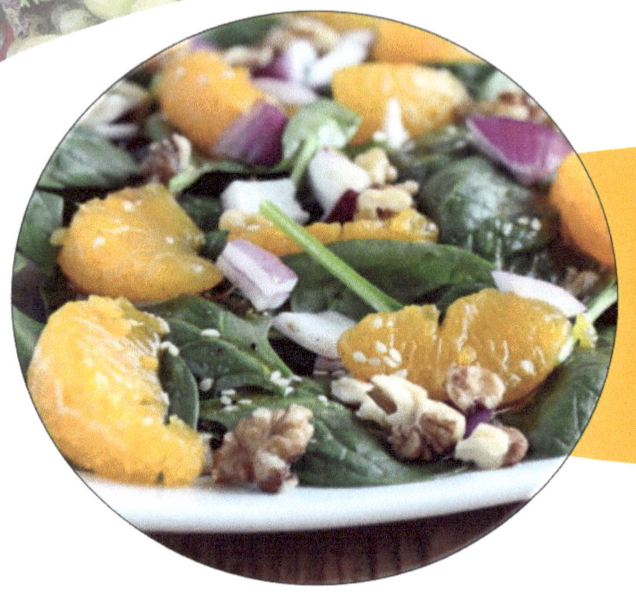

Lunch (Part 1)

Garden Salad Ingredients:

- 3 cups organic spinach and green leaf lettuce
- ½ cup cooked garbanzo beans
- ½ cup raw tomatoes
- 1 raw organic cucumber
- ¼ cup red onions
- ½ cup mandarin orange slices
- 2 tbl sp raw walnuts or sunflower seeds

Asian Vinaigrette Dressing

- 1/3 cup olive, avocado or peanut oil
- 2 tbl sp Rice vinegar or lemon juice
- 1 teaspoon gluten free, non gmo soy sauce
- 1/2 teaspoon sesame oil

Directions: Chop salad ingredients up and place in large bowl then mix dressing together and pour on top of salad. Serve with a bowl of lentil soup.

Lentil Soup

Lunch (Part 2)

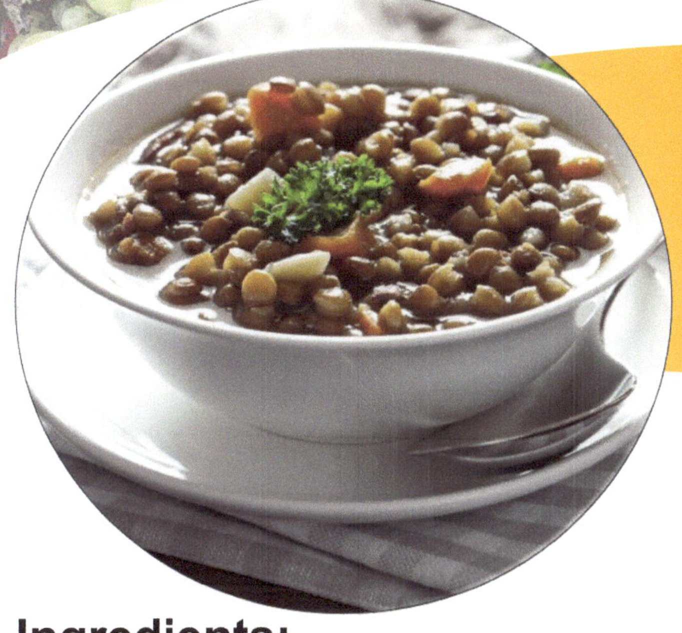

Ingredients:

- 1/2 lb. green or red lentils
- 1/2 Cup Wild rice, rinsed well
- 3 Large onions
- 4 Large stalks of celery
- 3 carrots diced
- 2 cloves garlic
- 2 tbl sp organic coconut oil
- 1 teaspoon low sodium herbal seasoning
- 1 teaspoon dried cumin or 1 drop cumin essential oil
- 1 teaspoon thyme or 1 drop of thyme essential oil
- 1 Quart vegetable broth (no MSG)
- 1 small can of tomato soup (BPA free)
- 2 teaspoon red wine vinegar

Directions:

- Cover lentils and rice with boiling water and let sit for 15 min then drain. In large stock pot, sauté the onions and garlic with the coconut oil and seasonings until the vegetables are tender. Add the carrots and celery and sauté another 5-10 minutes. Add the vegetables broth, tomato sauce and lentils. Bring to a boil, reduce heat and simmer 1 hour. Add vinegar and serve a bowl with salad.

Pico De Gallo & Chips

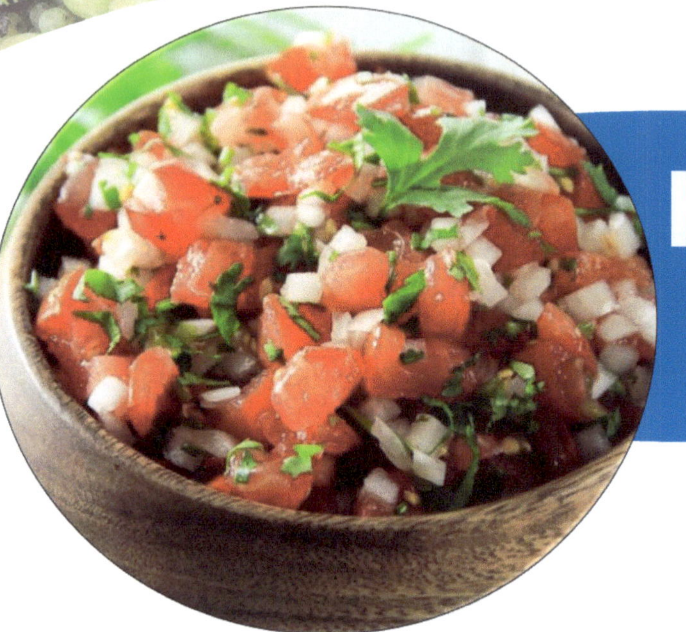

Healthy Snack

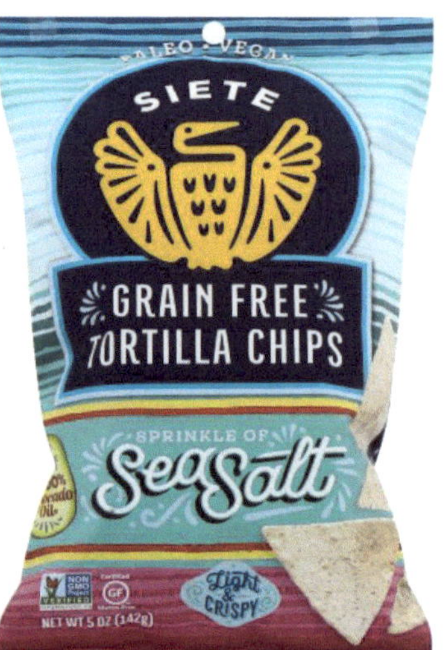

Pico de Gallo + Healthy Chips:

- 4 large organic roma tomatoes
- 2 small red onions (or 1 medium sized)
- 1 cup/10 cilantro stalks
- 2 drops lime essential oil
- Pinch of sea salt
- Pinch of garlic powder
- 1 cup of Baked Bean Crisps (Salt of the Earth)

Directions:

- Dice all veggies then mix together in a large bowl
- Add salt and lime oil then mix some more
- Eat with Baked (not fried) Bean Crisps or Casava Chips (Available at Sprouts, Costco, or other grocery stores)

Date Nut Balls

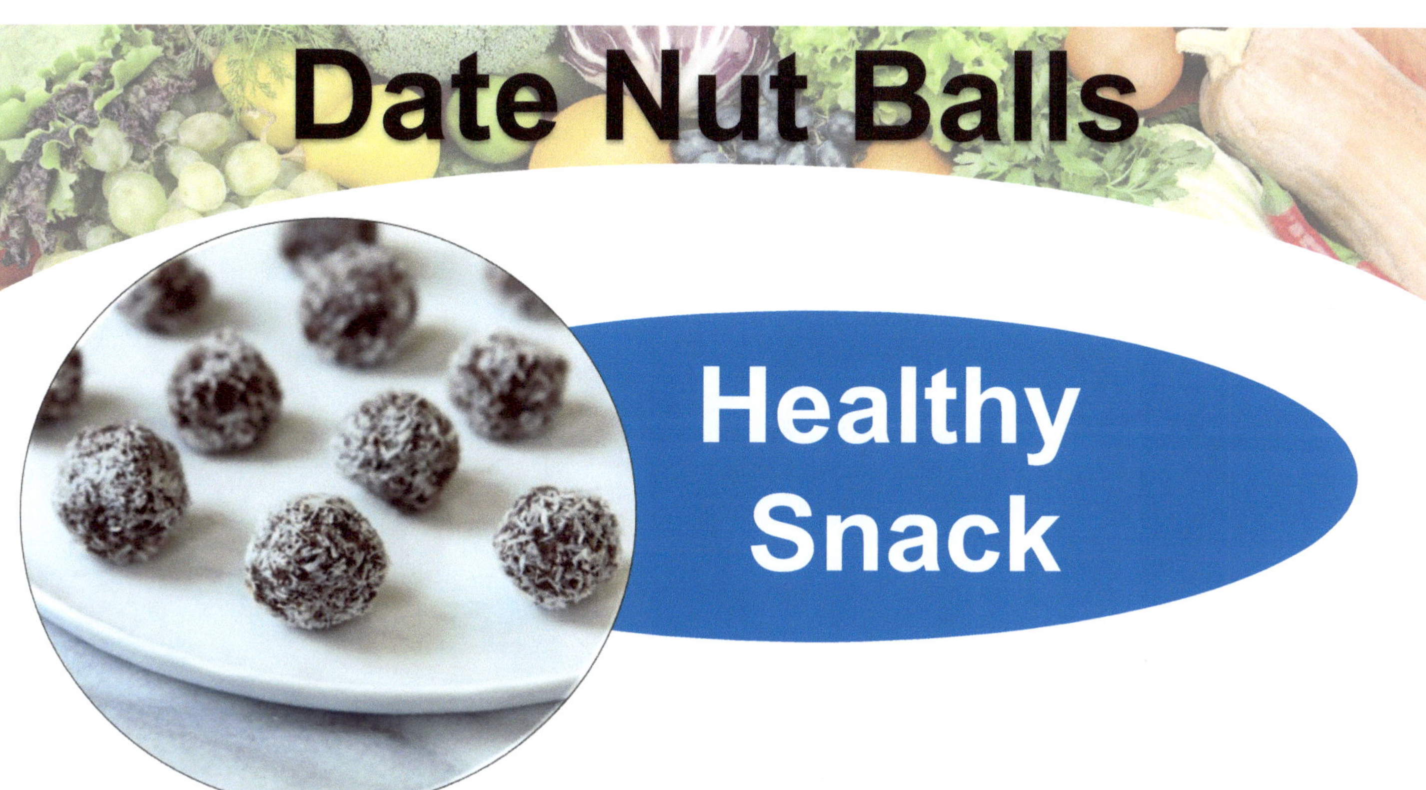

Healthy Snack

Ingredients:

- 1½ cup raw almonds (ground up in a food processor)
- 4–5 organic dates (pitted and cut up very finely)
- 2 Tbsp. raw sesame seeds
- 2 Tbsp. raw sunflower seeds
- 2 Tbsp. raw agave nectar
- ½ cup raw, no-sugar-added coconut flakes

Directions:

- **Step 1**: Work together everything except the reserved coconut flakes with your fingers until sticky*
- **Step 2**: Roll into balls
- **Step 3**: Roll into the coconut flakes on a plate
- **Step 4**: Put in fridge for about one hour before serving

*Note: Sometimes it has to sit for an hour or two before it will become sticky enough to roll into balls (depends on how many dates you use).

Savory Quinoa Salad

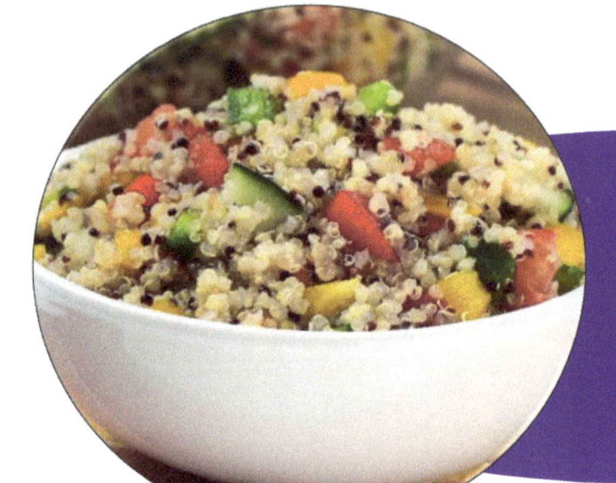

Dinner

Ingredients:

- 1 1/2 cup water
- 1 cup quinoa
- 2 medium bell peppers
- 1 small onion
- 1 1/2 teaspoon curry powder
- 1/4 cup cilantro
- 1 lime (Juiced)
- 1/4 cup almonds (Sliced)
- 1/2 cup carrots (Chopped)
- 1/2 cup cranberries (Dried)
- 1/8 teaspoon sea salt
- 1/8 teaspoon ground black pepper

Directions:

1.) Bring the water to a boil over high heat in a saucepan, then pour in the quinoa, cover with a lid, and continue to simmer over low heat until the water has been absorbed for about 15 to 20 minutes
2.) Once the quinoa is cooked, pour into a mixing bowl, and chill in the refrigerator for about 30 minutes
3.) Once chilled, stir in the red bell pepper, yellow bell pepper, red onion, curry powder, cilantro, lime juice, sliced almonds, carrots, and cranberries
4.) Season to taste with salt and pepper

Vegetable Stir Fry

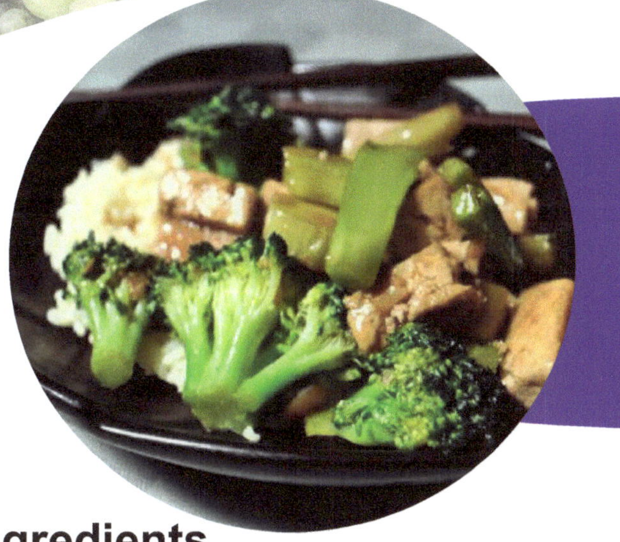

Ingredients

- ½ cup water
- 3 cups fresh cut broccoli
- 1 diced red bell pepper
- 1 diced onion
- ½ clove minced garlic
- 1 tablespoon minced ginger (or 1 drop doTERRA ginger oil)
- 1 tablespoon sesame seed oil
- ¼ black pepper
- 3 tablespoons Braggs liquid aminos
- 1 package of cubed tofu
- 2 minced green onions

Rice Replacement

- ½ cup red/orange lentils
- 1 cup millet
- 3 cups water

Directions:

- Soak the red/orange lentils and millet for at least 8 hours and cook on med-high heat until it comes to a boil then cook on low for 20 mins then shut off heat for 20 mins and let it steam cook
- Lightly sauté all the other ingredients together in a large pan for 20-30 mins until the broccoli is softer, but still semi- crisp. Serve over the Rice Replacement for more protein and fiber. Serves 4-6 people.

Purple Cabbage Salad

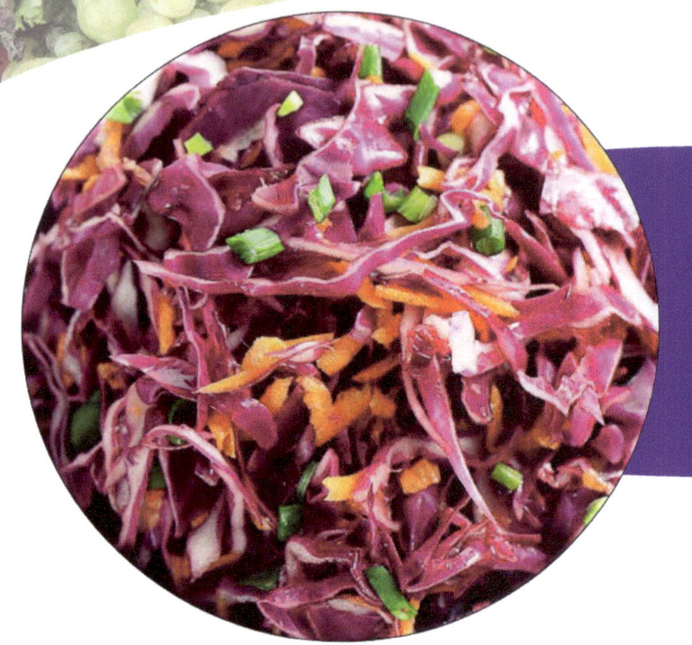

Dinner

Ingredients

- 2 Cups shredded green cabbage
- 2 Cups shredded purple cabbage
- 1 Cup shredded carrots
- ¼ Cup green onions
- 1/4 Cup golden raisins
- 1/4 Cup raw pumpkin seeds

Dressing:

- 2 Tbl sp real maple syrup
- 2 Tbl sp extra virgin olive oil
- 2 Tbl sp raw red wine vinegar
- 1 clove chopped garlic (or pre-chopped in jar)

Directions:

- Toss salad ingredients in a large bowl and pour dressing over and mix up well
- Enjoy with a healthy dessert!

Chocolate Avocado Pudding

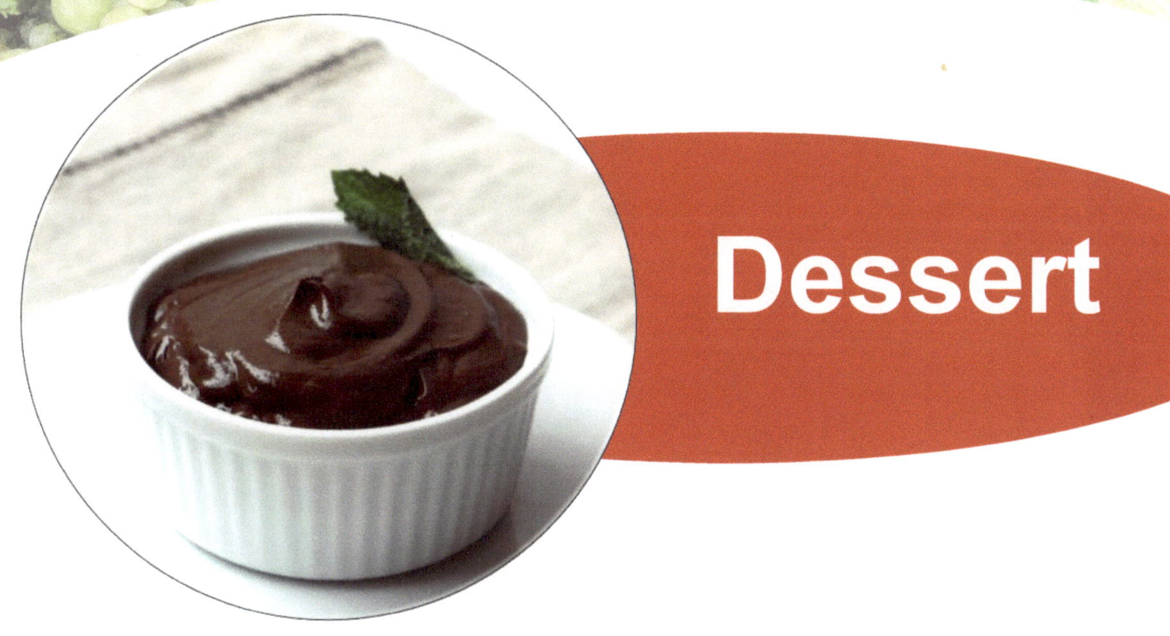

Dessert

Ingredients
- 6 avocados
- 1/2 cup raw agave
- 3/4 cup organic and raw cacao
- 2 drops cinnamon or cassia essential oil
- 1/2 scoop plant based protein powder (Orgain)
- 1 cup vanilla coconut milk (or vanilla almond milk)
- Pinch of sea salt

Directions:
- Blend all contents in a high powered blender until one texture is formed.
- Helps to have a cake spatula to mix in between blendings
- Serve a small bowl (1/4 cup) with ¼ cup cut up organic strawberries or raspberries
- Refrigerate the rest in a glass container with a lid on top

Black Bean Brownies

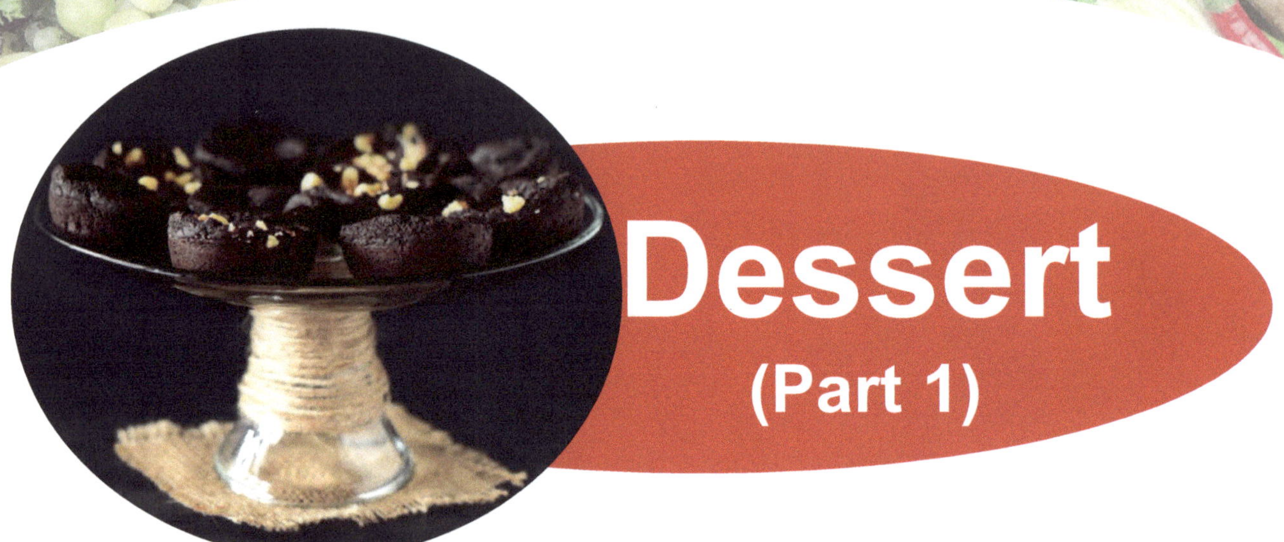

Ingredients

- 1, 15-oz. can (~ 1 3/4 cups) black beans (well rinsed and drained)
- 2 large *flax eggs* (2 heaping tablespoons flaxseed meal + 6 tablespoons water)
- 3 tablespoons coconut oil (melted)
- 3/4 cup organic cocoa powder
- 1/4 teaspoon sea salt
- 1 teaspoon pure organic vanilla extract
- 1/2 cup agave nectar
- 1 1/2 teaspoon baking powder

- *Optional toppings*: crush walnuts, pecans, or dairy-free semisweet chocolate chips, 1 drop of doTERRA lemon essential oil (per muffin)

***Note:** See next page for directions…
**Supports energy, digestion, and weight loss goals when you eat 1-2 per meal as the dessert

Black Bean Brownies

Directions

1. Preheat oven to 350 degrees F (176 C)
2. Lightly grease a 12-slot standard size muffin pan with coconut oil
3. Prepare flax eggs by combining flax and water in the bowl of the food processor and pulsing for 30 seconds
4. Add remaining ingredients (besides walnuts or other toppings) and puree until smooth (for about 3 mins)
5. If the batter appears too thick, add a tablespoon or two of water and pulse again
6. Evenly distribute the batter into the muffin tin and smooth the tops with a spoon or your finger.
7. Bake for 20-26 minutes or until the tops are dry and the edges start to pull away from the sides.
8. Remove from oven and let cool for 30 minutes before removing from pan. They will be tender, so remove gently with a fork. The insides are meant to be very fudgy since they dry up in storage
9. Store in an airtight container for up to a few days. Refrigerate to keep longer.

DIY Juicing Recipe

1.) Starting Veggies (Choose a cup of each)

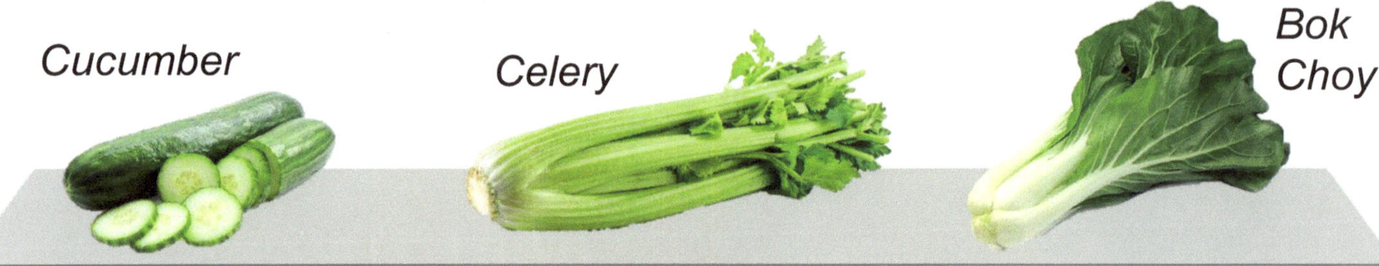

2.) Green Leafies (Choose a handful of each)

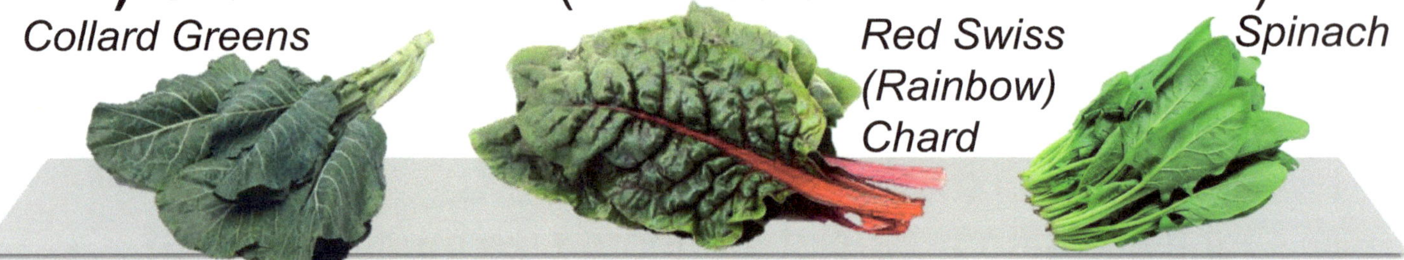

3.) Natural Sweeteners (Choose 1-2 options below

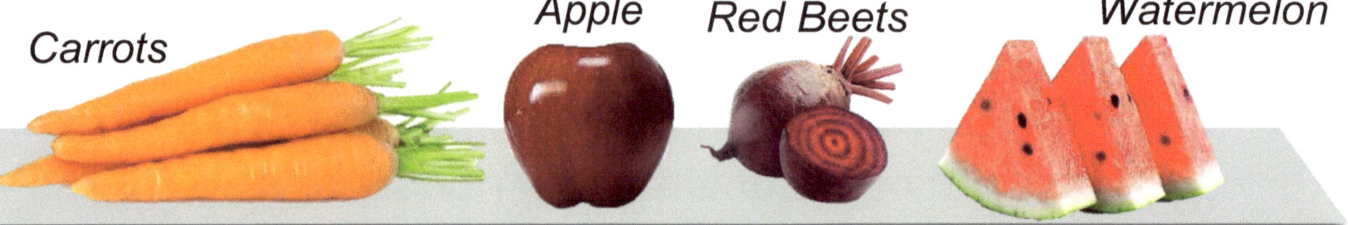

4.) Alkalizers (Choose 1-2) 5.) Detoxifiers (Choose 1)

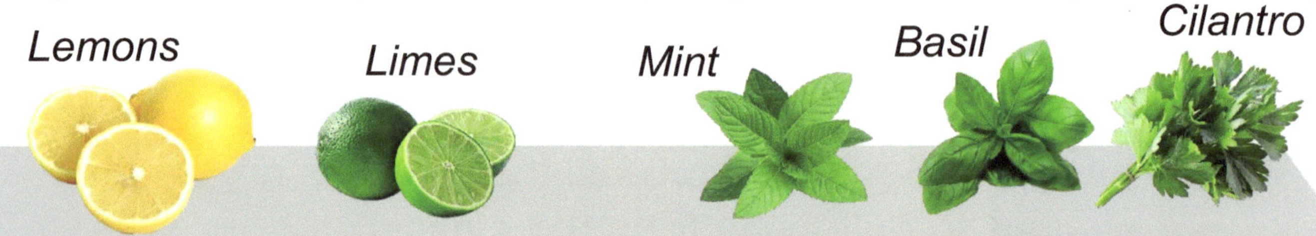

Directions: Juice starting veggies, remove tough stems from collards and chard then juice. Juice sweeteners and keep in mind apples are better for flavor but beets dominate in color. Next, juice the alkalizers without the peel for less bitterness. Finally juice herbs by tightly packing them down, but know that a little bit goes a long way (especially mint).

Best Practices: Add alkaline water to your juice to extend it's life and drink at room temperature since it's better for digestion. Supplementing your meals or doing a juice fast for 1-3 days is a good starting point.

Slim Down Juice Recipe

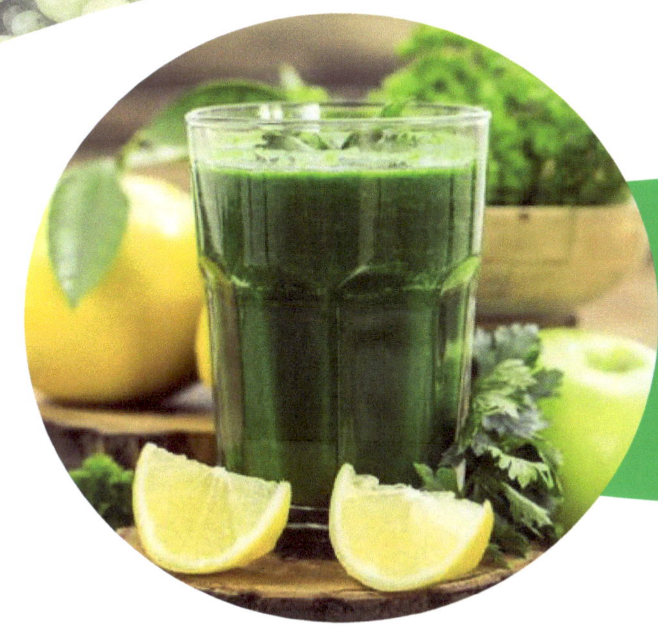

Juice

Ingredients:

- 1 organic cucumber
- 2 large carrots
- 1 organic fuji or red delicious apple
- 4 celery stalks
- 1 small piece of ginger (or 1 drop doTERRA Ginger oil)
- 1 lemon
- 1 cup of fresh parsley

Directions:

1. Add all ingredients in a vegetable juicer
2. Gently mix the juice and consume immediately

*Serves 2, Time: 10-15 mins
**Supports energy, digestion, and weight loss

Lemon Detox Mocktail

1. Lemon essential oil*: Detoxes liver, kidney, lymphatic system, and bladder. Energizes. (6 drops)

2. Lime essential oil*: Promotes a healthy immune system, purifies body, adds flavor (6 drops)

3. Basil essential oil*: Antioxidants, improves immune system, and helps with energy (2 drops)

4. Ginger essential oil*: Helps with digestion and feelings of queasiness (2 drops)

5. Organic & Raw Agave Nectar: Less processed and lower on glycemic index (4 tbl sp**)

6. Organic Trace Minerals: Detoxes cells, provides energy, and fills in gap from what's not in food since soils are depleted (4 droppers full)

7. Ionized, Micro-clustered, Alkaline Water: Has antioxidants, hydrates cells by passing through membrane, promotes wellness, BPA free (1 gallon)

Directions: Combine ingredients above in a large 1 gallon glass pitcher and stir. Drink 8 oz when you wake up since body is dehydrated and drink ½ your body weight in ounces throughout the day (e.g. 160 lbs drinks 80 ounces, **Note:** 1 gallon = 128 ounces). Drink more when working out and sweating or when out in the sun for more than 15 mins.

*Only Certified Pure Therapeutic Grade (CPTG) essential oils
**Not recommended for the morning since blood sugar is already low

How To Use Lemon Oil

Lemon Oil Substitution Guideline

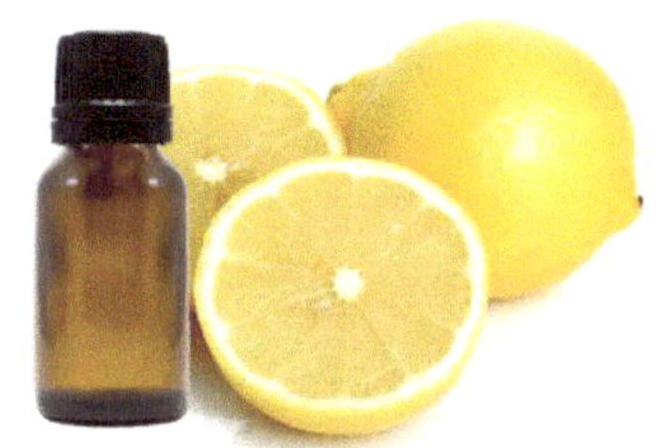

1 drop of lemon oil can be substitute for 1 teaspoon of citrus zest. If your recipe calls for the zest from 1 lemon, then you can use 3-5 drops of the lemon essential oil instead.* This will add flavor and health benefits.

Health Benefits

Lemon oil cleanses and purifies the air and surfaces, naturally cleanses the body, and promotes a more positive mood.

Primary Uses

- **Aromatic:** Use 3-5 drops in a 4 hour diffuser
- **Internal:** Dilute one drop in 4 ounces of water
- **Topical:** Apply 1-2 drops on palms of hands, rub together, then breathe in (avoid eyes)

Lemon Oil In Recipes

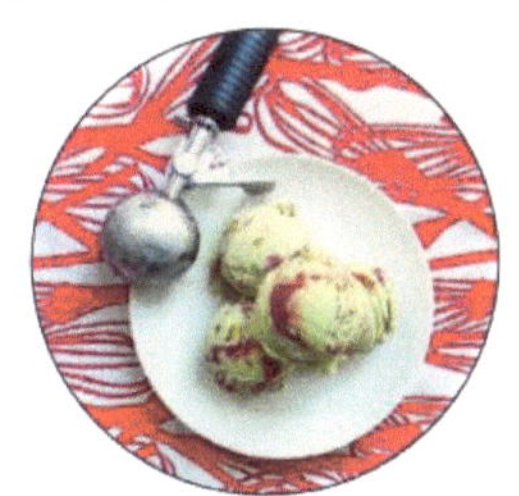

Strawberry Avocado Ice Cream

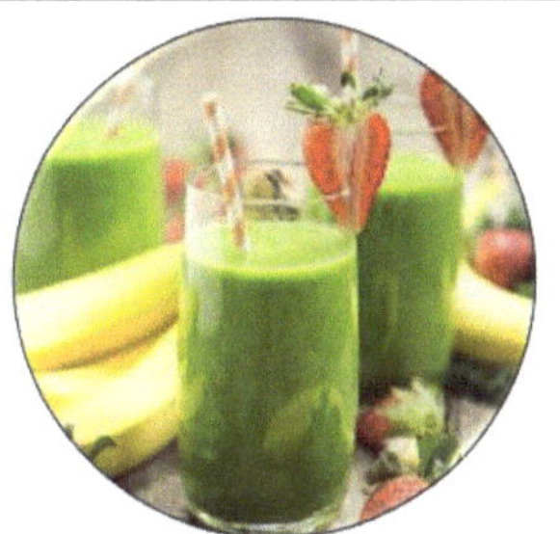

Green Smoothies

Coconut Lemon Bars

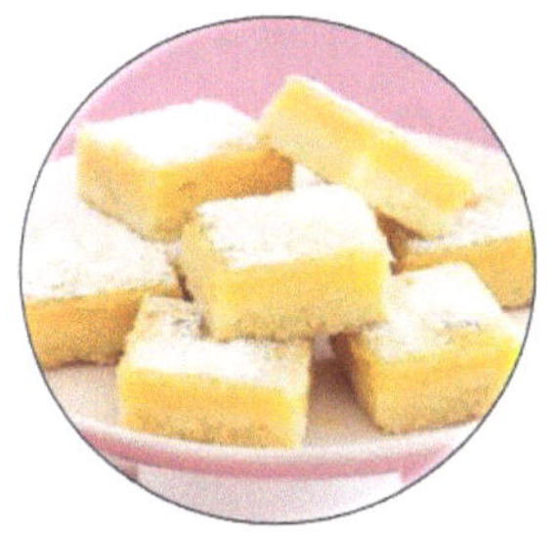

Lemon Tarragon Salad Dressing

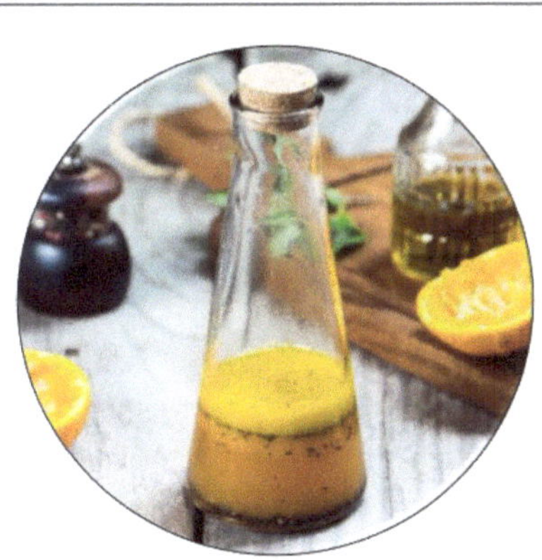

Ingredients:
- 1 teaspoon dried tarragon
- 1 teaspoon dried basil leaves
- 1 cup extra virgin olive oil
- 1/3 cup apple cider vinegar
- Dash of black pepper
- Dash of sea salt
- Dash of red pepper
- 6 drops of lemon essential oil*

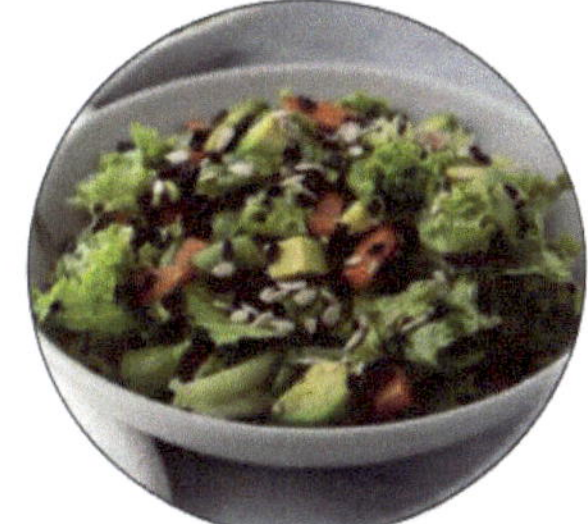

Directions: Mix ingredients well and drizzle onto homemade salad. Keep unused portion in fridge.

*Only use Certified Pure essential oils that are 3rd party tested for internal use.
**Disclaimer: These statements have not been evaluated by the FDA and are not intended to diagnose, treat or cure any disease. Results may vary depending on starting point, goals and effort.

How To Use Peppermint Oil

Peppermint Oil Substitution Guideline

1 drop of peppermint essential oil equals about 1 teaspoon of dried peppermint leaves or 1 tablespoon of fresh mint leaves.

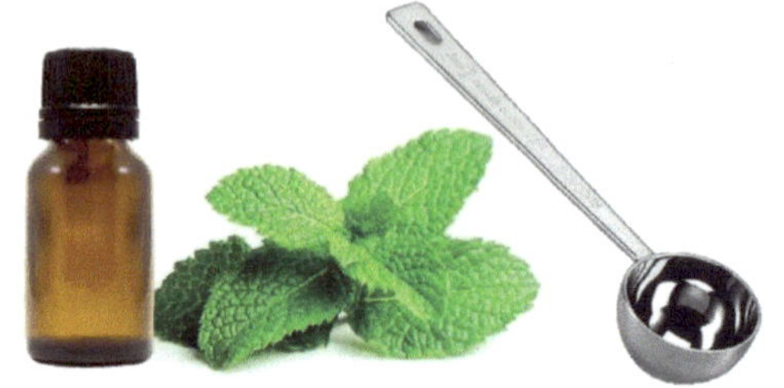

Health Benefits

Helps increase focus and alertness, promotes healthy digestive function, and reduces head tension

Primary Uses

- **Aromatic:** Use 3-5 drops in a 4 hour diffuser
- **Internal:** Dilute two drops in 8 ounces of water
- **Topical:** Add 2-3 drops to reflex points with fractionated coconut oil

Peppermint Oil In Recipes

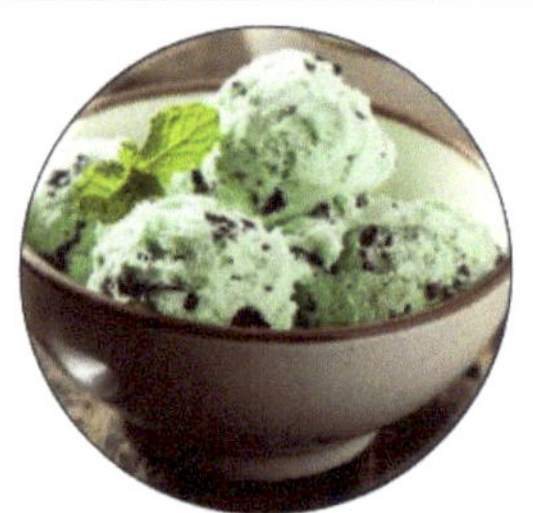

Homemade Mint Chocolate Chip Ice Cream

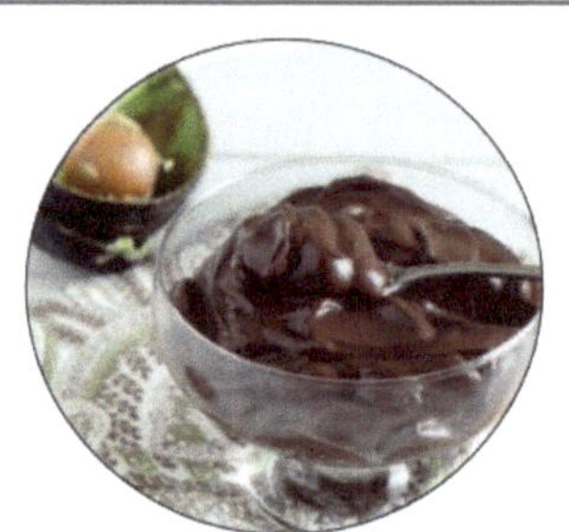

Mint Chocolate Avocado Pudding

Mint Black Bean Brownies

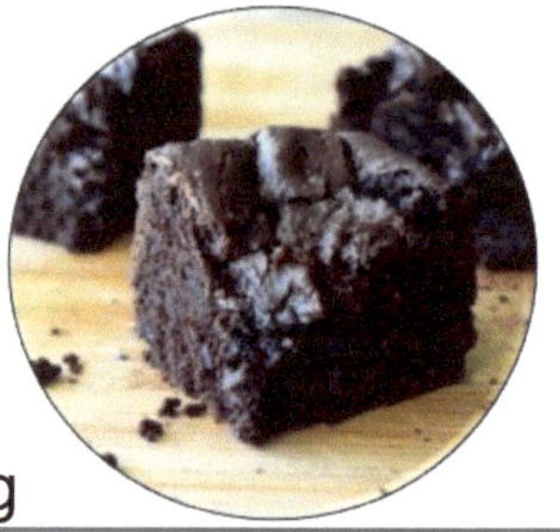

Mint Chocolate Smoothie

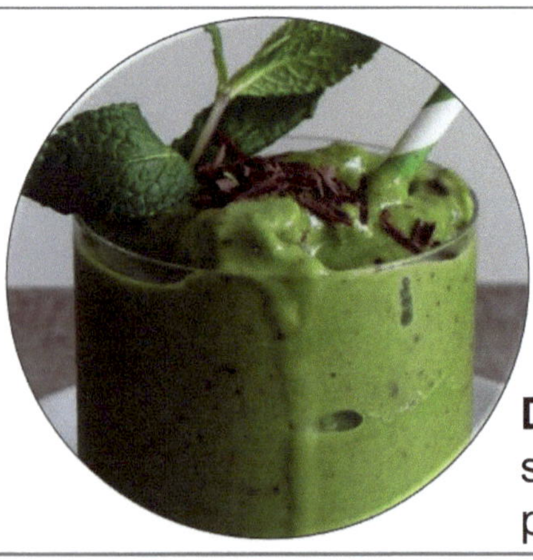

Ingredients:
- 2 cups vanilla coconut milk (or almond milk)
- 1 ½ cup ice
- 2 cups organic baby spinach
- 1 drop peppermint oil
- 2 bananas (peeled)
- 1 scoop plant based protein powder (Orgain)
- Organic and raw cacao nibs

Directions: In a high-speed blender, blend coconut milk, ice, spinach, & peppermint for 30 seconds. Add bananas, protein powder, & blend until smooth. Mix in nibs or add on top.

How To Use Oregano Oil

Oregano Oil Substitution Guideline

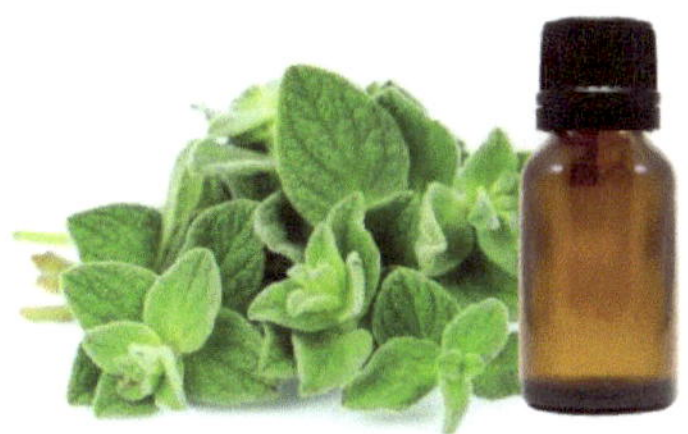

Start with dipping a toothpick in the oil bottle and stirring it in the mixture and then add more to taste as needed. Typically 1 drop of oregano oil equals 1 teaspoon of dried oregano herb.

Health Benefits

Powerful cleansing and purifying agent, supports a healthy immune system, kicks bad guys out of the gut

Primary Uses

- **Aromatic:** Use 3-5 drops in a 4 hour diffuser
- **Internal:** Place 3-5 drops in an empty veggie capsule and drink with water and food
- **Topical:** Dilute 1-2 drops with fractionated coconut oil and use on reflex points

Oregano Oil In Recipes

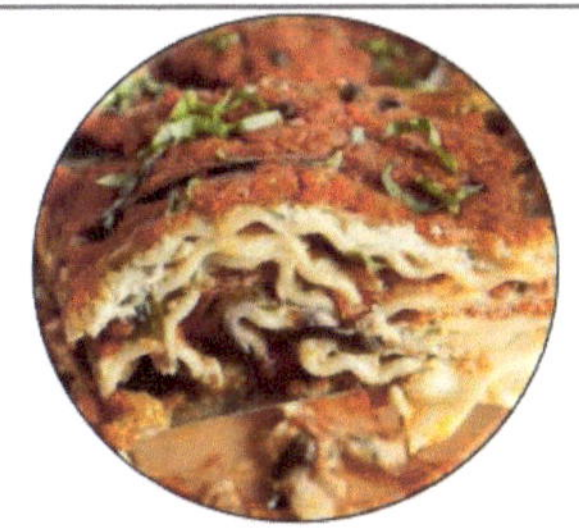

Homemade Vegan Lasagna

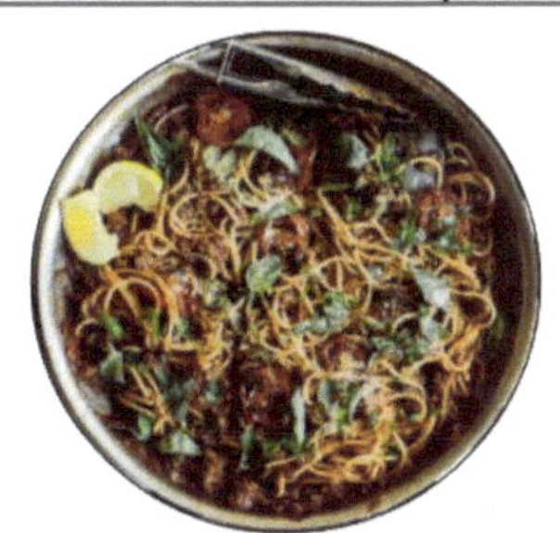

Gluten Free Spaghetti

Minestrone Soup

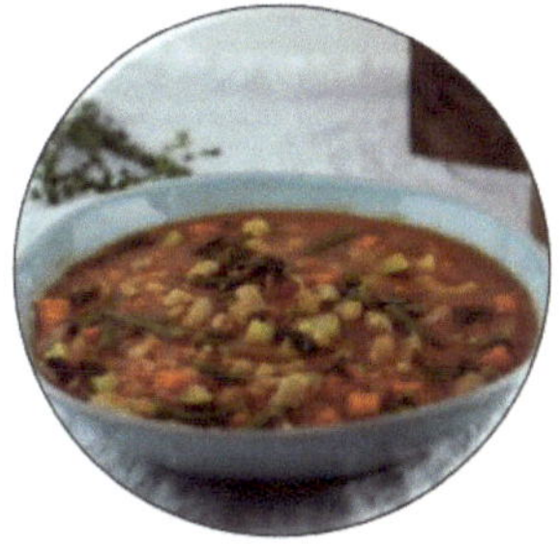

Homemade Pizza/Marinara Sauce

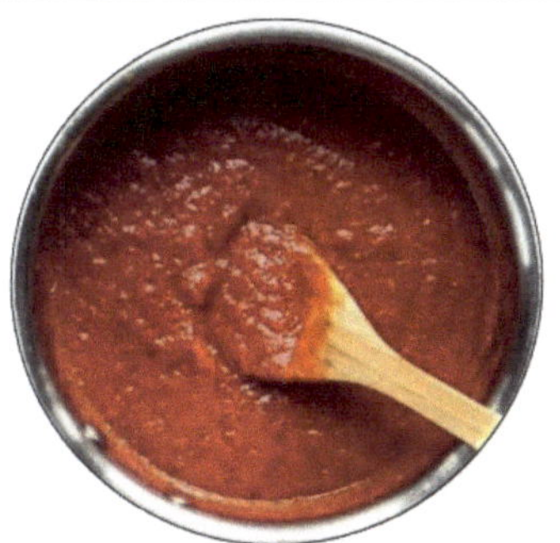

Ingredients:
- 1 can (27 fl. oz/796 mL) organic diced tomatoes
- 2 cloves fresh garlic
- 1 tablespoons onion powder
- 1 drop oregano oil
- 1 drop thyme oil
- 1 drop basil oil
- 1/2 teaspoon sea salt (add more to taste)

Directions: Blend all ingredients for 30 seconds, place in pot and cook on medium heat for 30 mins until it boils, then transfer to a jar and let cool before putting in fridge

Whole Food Vitamins

The 3 Fold Problem

1. Our soils have been depleted of vitamins, minerals, and trace minerals causing our plants to be void of them and then causing us to be void of them
2. Most vitamins in grocery stores and online are made in labs and contain synthetic ingredients (i.e. no absorption & cheapest)
3. Other vitamins in stores and online are made with rock derived minerals (i.e. low absorption & cheaper)

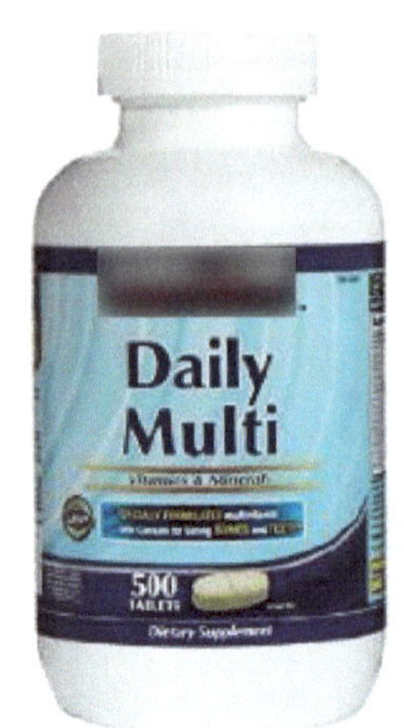

The Natural Solution

Using wholefood vitamins and minerals allows you to:
- Have higher cellular absorption
- Fill in the nutrient gap missing in your diet
- Ingredient quality matters

What To Look For

You want to look for a natural vitamin and mineral supplement with whole food nutrients that are bound to a *glycoprotein matrix* to enhance their cellular absorption within your body.

Health Benefits

These nutrients:
- Support healthy cell, tissue, organ, and body system function
- Helps repair free radical damage

Hot Pink Smoothie Recipe (Increases Vitamin Absorption)

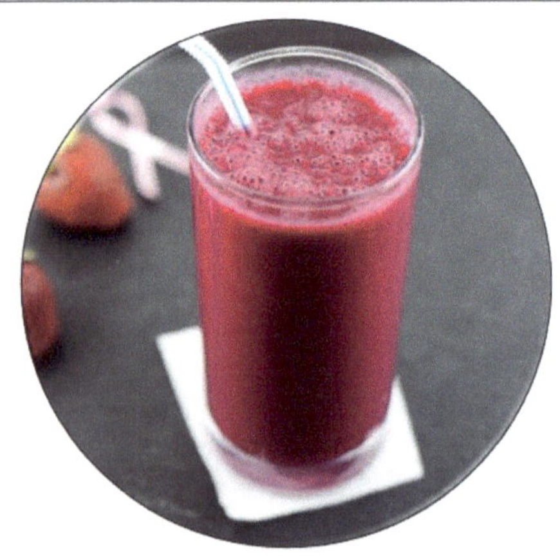

Ingredients:
- 1 ½ cup coconut liquid (raw or from can)
- 1 large carrot (cleaned and cut into 3 pieces)
- ¼ of medium sized beet (cleaned and raw)
- ¼ cup cashews (soaked overnight and drained)
- ¼ cup chopped dates (pitted)
- 2 teaspoon pure vanilla
- 12 frozen and organic strawberries
- 1 scoop plant based protein powder (Orgain)

Directions: In a high-speed blender, blend everything except strawberries and protein powder for 30 seconds. Add remaining ingredients and blend until smooth. Makes 4 cups of hotness

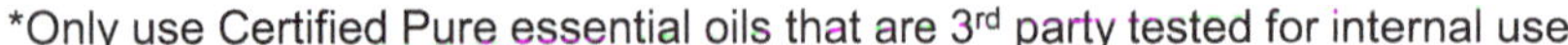

*Only use Certified Pure essential oils that are 3rd party tested for internal use.
**Disclaimer: These statements have not been evaluated by the FDA and are not intended to diagnose, treat or cure any disease. Results may vary depending on starting point, goals and effort.

Antioxidant Supplements

Problem #1

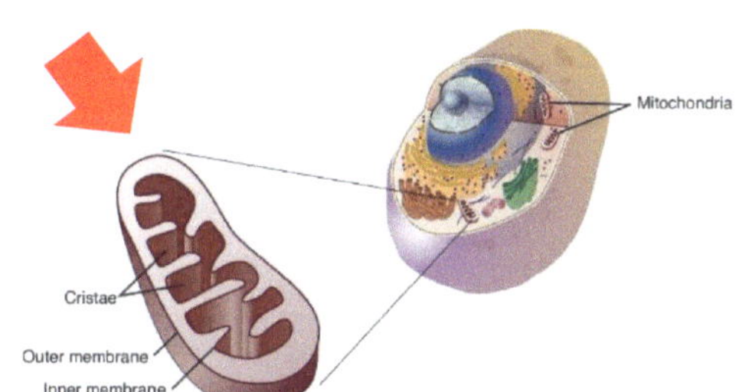

- **Mitochondria** are the little engines of your cells and as you get older, the quantity and efficiency of these little motors decreases.
- This results in **less energy** available for your body.

Problem #2

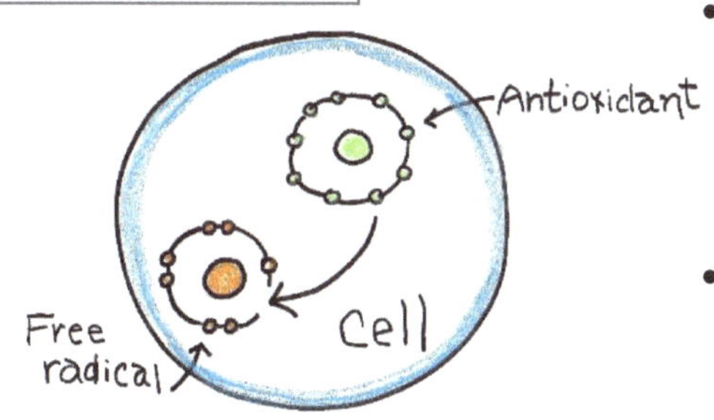

- **Free radicals** are unstable molecules that can start a damaging chain reaction of cellular oxidation contributing to premature aging and inflammation in your body.
- **Free radicals** are a toxic byproduct of breathing, metabolism of food, pollution, smoking, sunlight, and exposure to radiation (they can't be avoided!)

The Natural Solution

Polyphenols & Antioxidants from a natural and high quality supplement source

Health Benefits

- Neutralize free radicals from causing "domino effect"
- Protect DNA and mitochondria from damage
- Increase energy on a cellular level without stimulants

Savory V8 Smoothie (Enhances Antioxidant Benefits)

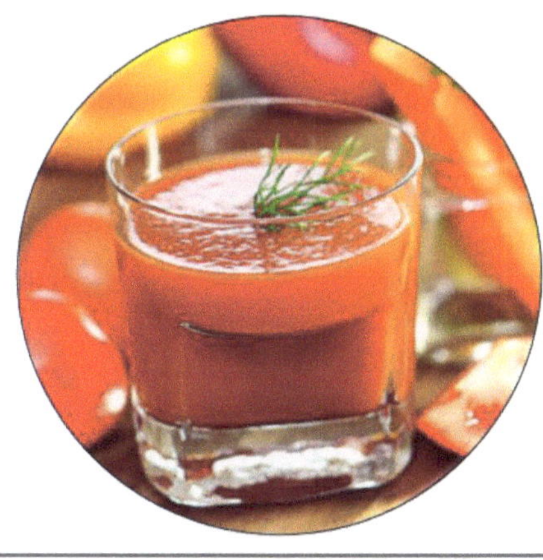

Ingredients:

- 2 cups alkaline water
- 1 handful spinach
- 1 kale leaf (with stem)
- 1 carrot
- 2 tomatoes
- 1 stalk of green onion
- 2 celery stalks
- ½ cucumber
- 1 cup ice
- Juice of 1 lemon
- Basil leaves (to taste)
- Cilantro leaves (to taste)
- Sea Salt (to taste)

Directions: In a high-speed blender, blend water, ice, & greens for 30 seconds. Add rest of veggies, and sea salt then blend until smooth. Choose all organic ingredients for optimal quality.

*Only use Certified Pure essential oils that are 3rd party tested for internal use.
**Disclaimer: These statements have not been evaluated by the FDA and are not intended to diagnose, treat or cure any disease. Results may vary depending on starting point, goals and effort.

Omega 3 Supplements

The 3 Fold Problem

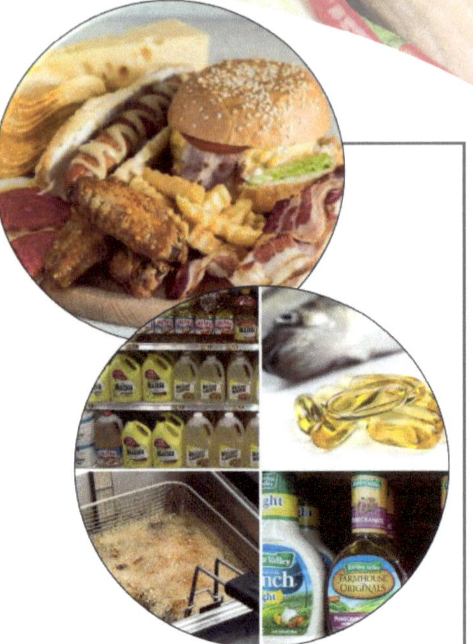

1. The Standard American Diet (spells S-A-D or SAD) of processed foods is high in Omega-6's, destroys your endocrine system, and causes internal inflammation.
2. Americans are Omega 3 deficient and most people get between 10:1 and 25:1 Omega 6's to Omega 3's. The ideal ratio is 1:1 and 4:1 Omega 6's to Omega 3's.
3. High Omega 6 ratios have been linked to depression, cancer, heart disease, stroke, asthma, lupus, diabetes, ADHD, and Alzheimer's.

The Natural Solution

You want to look for a Omega 3 supplement that contains essential fatty acids from clean sources where the
- Mercury has been filtered out
- Contains the antioxidant astaxanthin
- Has essential oils for extra support

Health Benefits

Omega-3 fatty acids are not produced by your body, but can help
- Support healthy joints & muscles
- Support Cardiovascular system
- Improve brain function
- Strengthen Immune system

Waterloupe Smoothie (Increases Benefits Of Omega 3's)

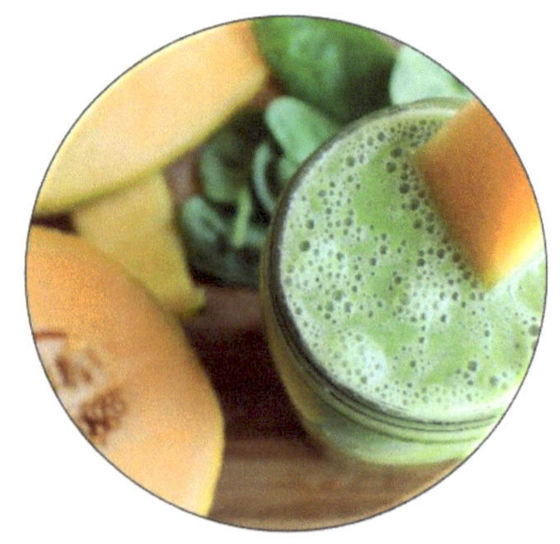

Ingredients:
- 2 cups vanilla coconut milk
- ½ cup ice
- 3 cups organic spinach
- 1 cup cantaloupe chunks
- 1 cup watermelon chunks
- 1 banana
- 1 scoop plant based protein powder (Orgain)

Directions: In a high-speed blender, blend coconut milk, ice, and spinach for 30 seconds. Add melons, banana, protein powder, and blend until smooth.

*Only use Certified Pure essential oils that are 3rd party tested for internal use.
**Disclaimer: These statements have not been evaluated by the FDA and are not intended to diagnose, treat or cure any disease. Results may vary depending on starting point, goals and effort.

Costco Shoppers Guide

> **GOAL:** Each time you shop, make sure you have foods from each of these categories below in your kitchen pantry. Greens are the most nutrient dense and low calorie option and should be a first choice!

❑ **Green Leafy Vegetables** (3-6 cups per day)
   Broccoli, kale, spinach, chard, collard greens, green leafy salad, brussel sprouts, bok-choy

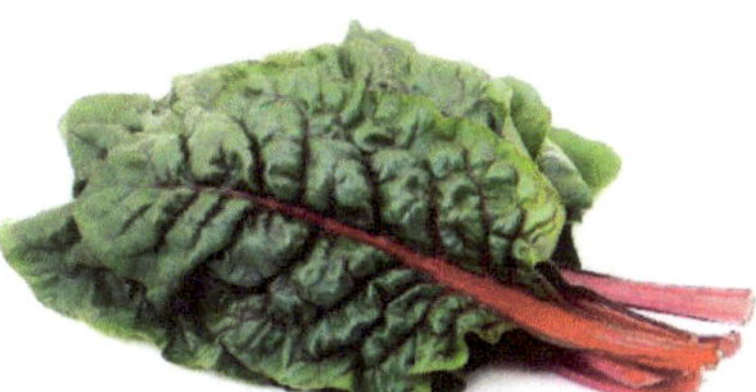

❑ **Other Vegetables** (3-4 cups per day)
   Beets, carrots, peppers, tomatoes, avocado, onions, fennel, asparagus, peas, artichokes

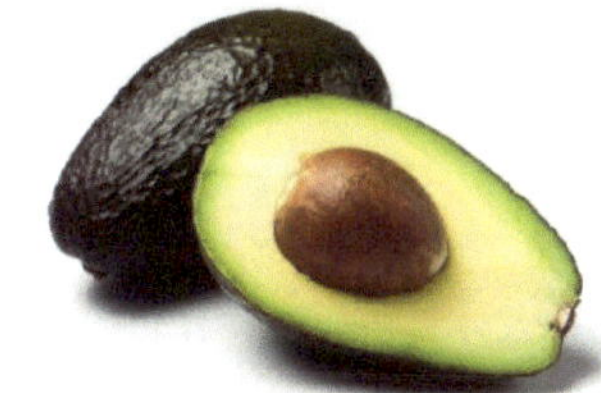

❑ **Fruits** (2-3 servings per day)
   Blueberries, cherries, strawberries, blackberries, raspberries, mangoes, bananas, apples, oranges, watermelon

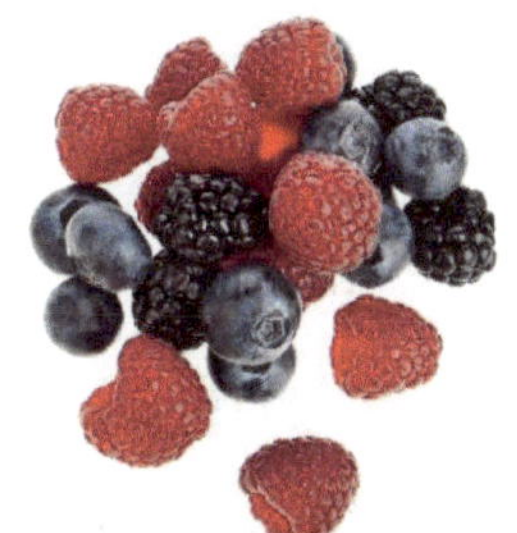

❑ **Legumes** (1-2 servings)
   Black, red, pinto, garbanzo, lentils, navy, cannellini, (any bean is good), plus tempeh or edamame
   (all soy products should be organic and non-GMO)

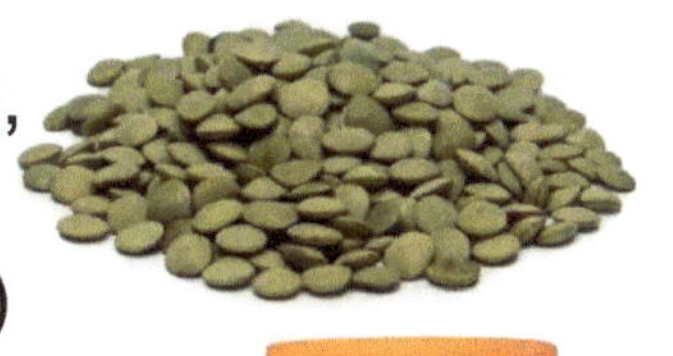

❑ **Healthy Oils** (1-2 tablespoons per day)
   Extra virgin olive oil, avocado oil, coconut oil, almond oil

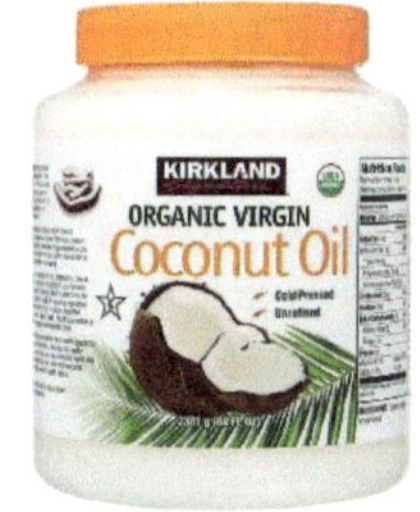

❑ **Nuts** (1-2 ounces per day)
   Almonds, pecans, walnuts, pistachios, hazelnuts, macadamia, brazil nuts (raw and unsalted are ideal)

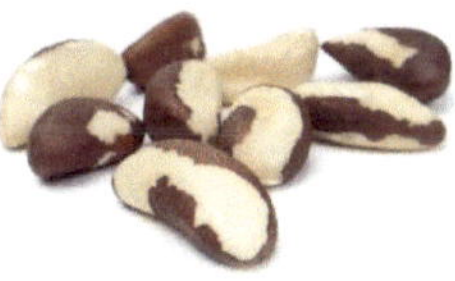

*Choose organic for thin skinned fruits and veggies to avoid pesticide and herbicide residue

Costco Shoppers Guide

Replace and Avoid These

GOAL: Each time you shop, be sure to avoid foods on this list below. These foods are either overly processed, acidic, or don't contribute to an environment of wellness in your body.

1.) Processed Fats

Don't buy foods with partially hydrogenated fats; think of this ingredient as embalming fluid. You also want to avoid vegetable, corn, soy, and canola oils since they are high in omega 6's and are inflammation causing.

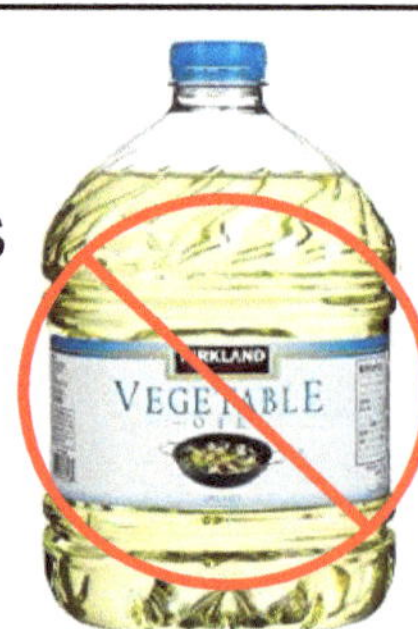

2.) Processed Meats

Don't buy foods made with nitrosamines, nitrites, or nitrates such as bacon, sandwich meats, sausage, pepperoni, ham, hot dogs, and deli meats. These chemical compounds are toxic and carcinogenic.

3.) Processed Sugars

Don't buy high fructose corn syrup, corn syrup, white sugar, corn starch, fruit juice, soda, diet soda, or sweet tea. These are void of fiber and excess calories are stored as fat. Diet or sugar free sodas contain aspartame or sucralose which are neurotoxins. Choose water, whole fruits, or agave nectar.

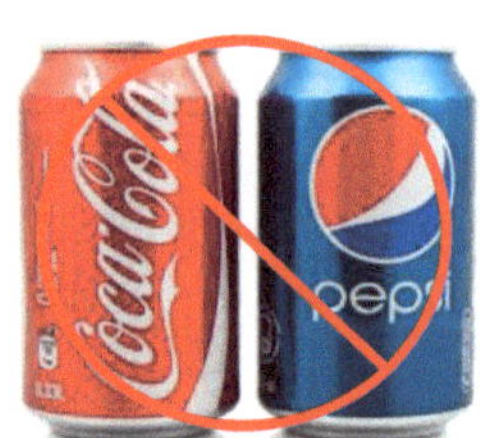

4.) Processed Carbs

Don't buy white rice, white pasta, white bread, corn flakes, white potatoes, french fries, potato chips, corn chips, wheat and corn tortillas. Choose bean chips, dehydrated fruits, millet, or quinoa instead.

*Disclaimer: These statements have not been evaluated by the FDA and are not intended to diagnose, treat or cure any disease. Results may vary depending on starting point, goals and effort.

Documentaries To Watch

Directions: Check off each documentary below that you watched on Amazon or Netflix over the next month to better support your first 30 days of the Green Smoothie Challenge.

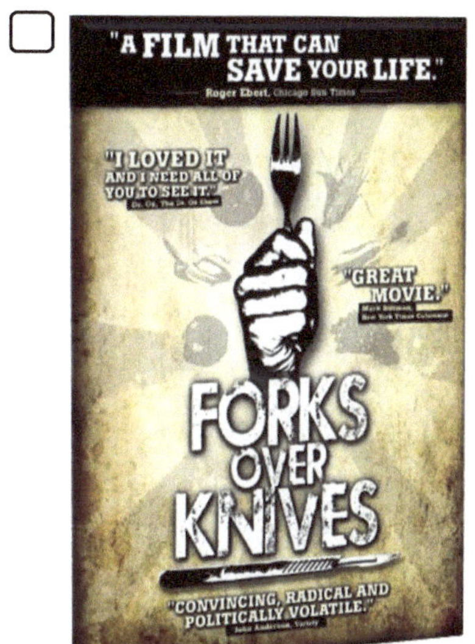

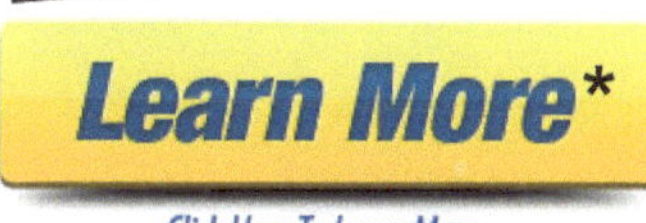

Click Here To Learn More...

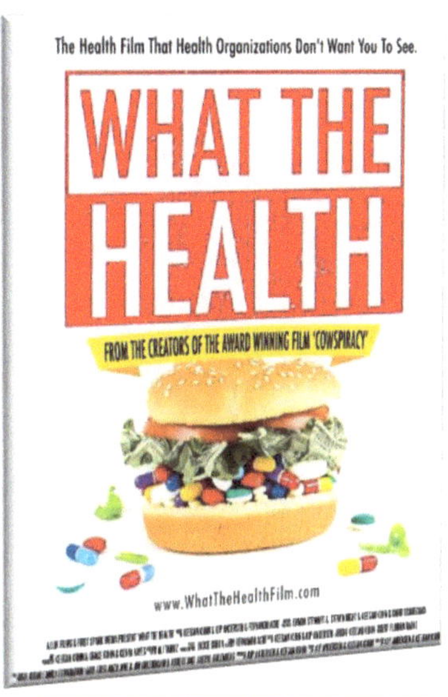

Click Here To Learn More...

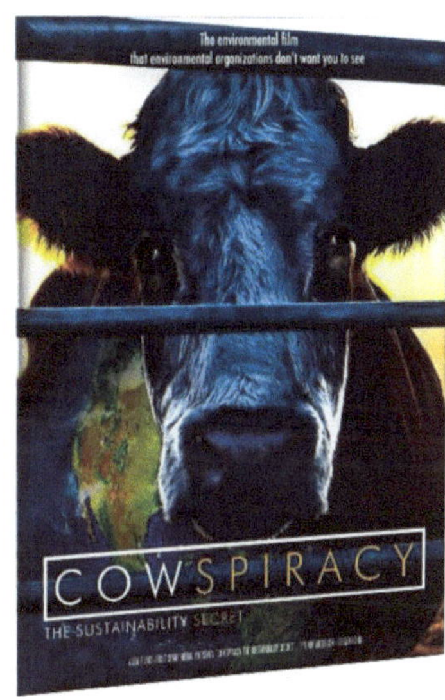

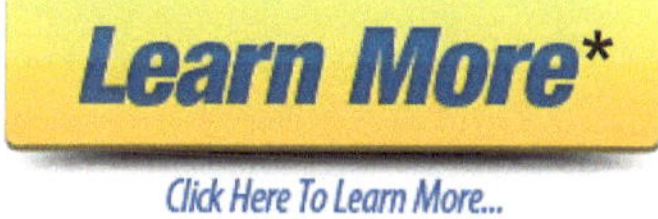

Click Here To Learn More...

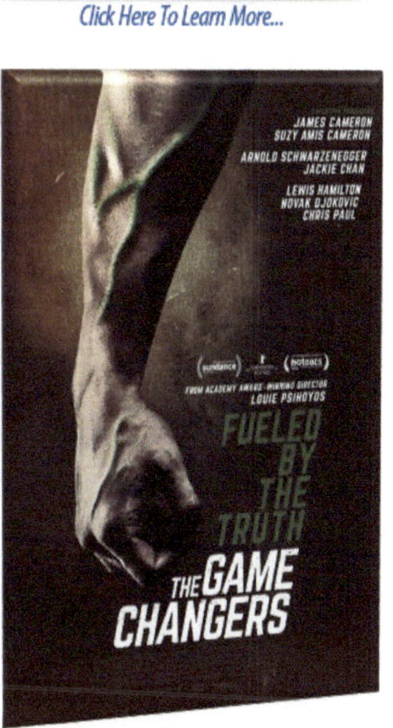

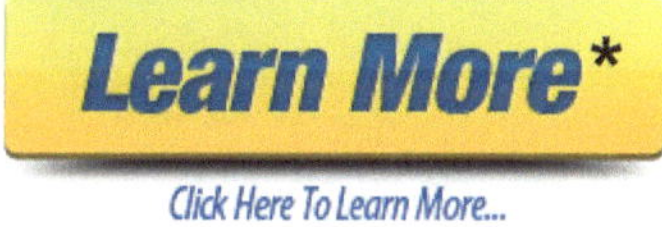

Click Here To Learn More...

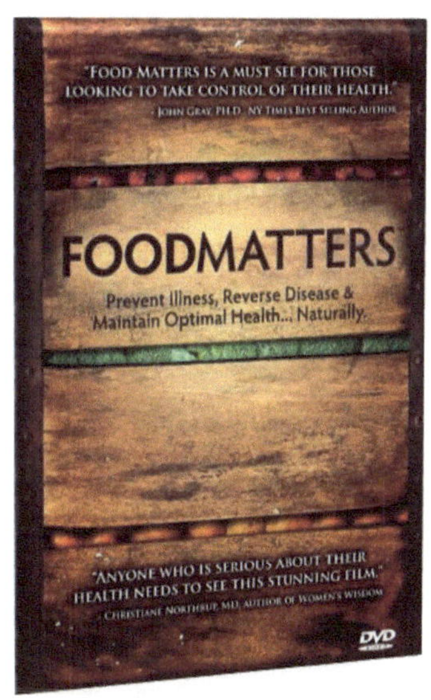

Click Here To Learn More...

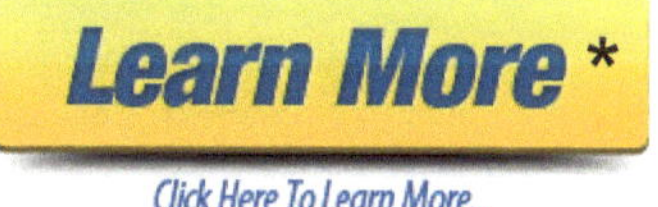

Click Here To Learn More...

*Clickable link available on ebook version of this page

Documentaries To Watch

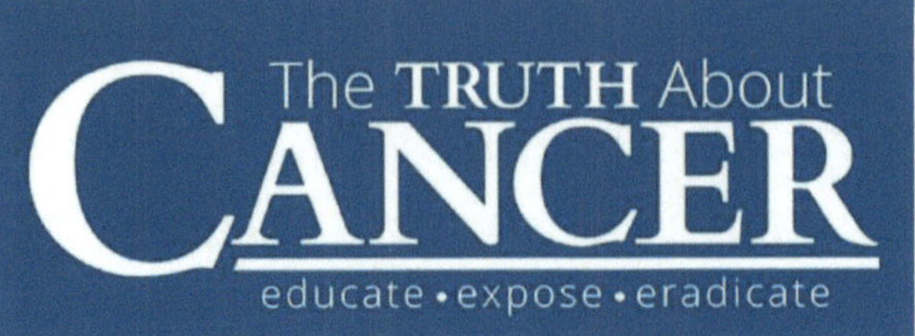

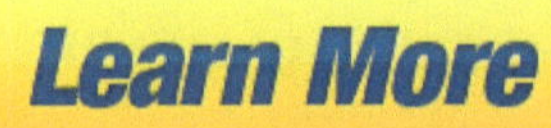

Click Here To Learn More...

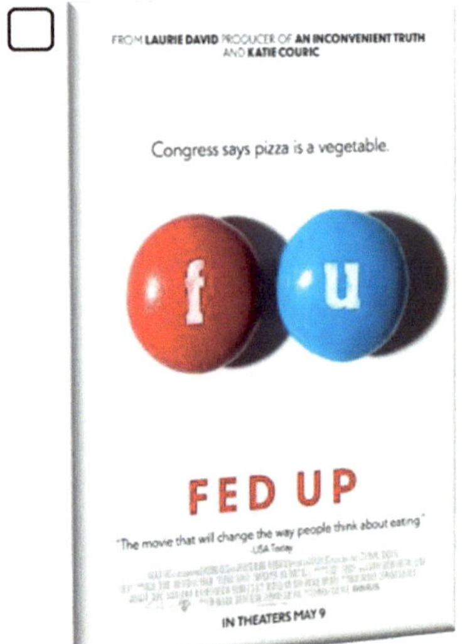

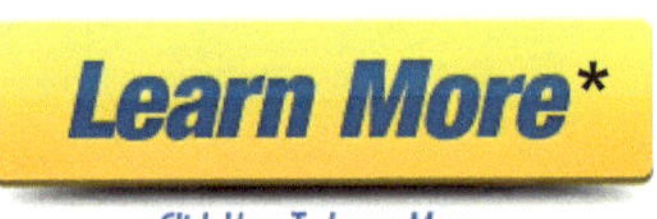

Click Here To Learn More...

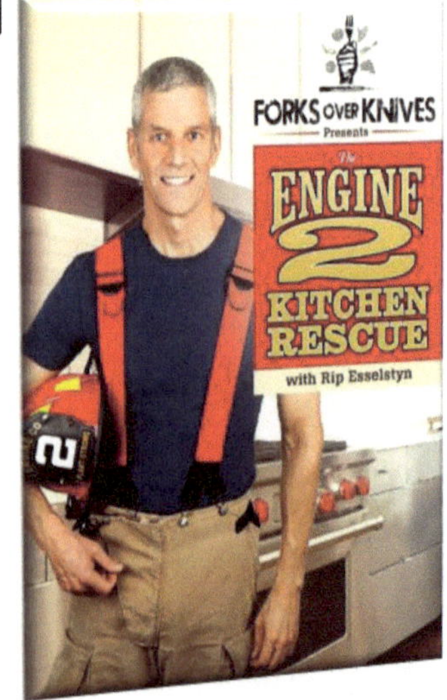

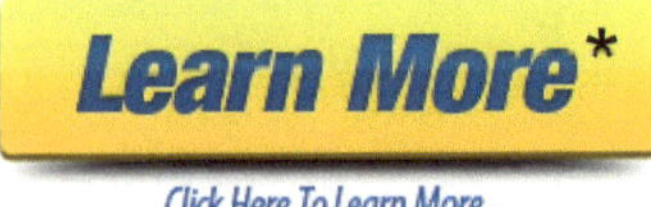

Click Here To Learn More...

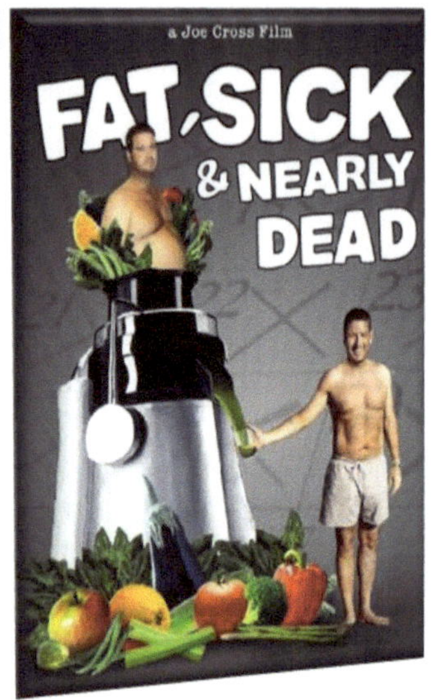

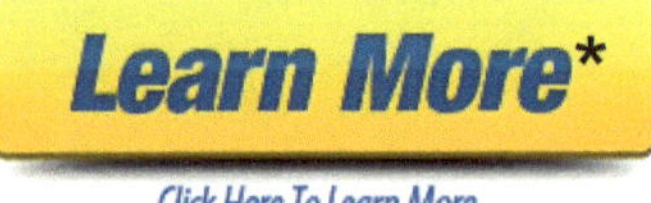

Click Here To Learn More...

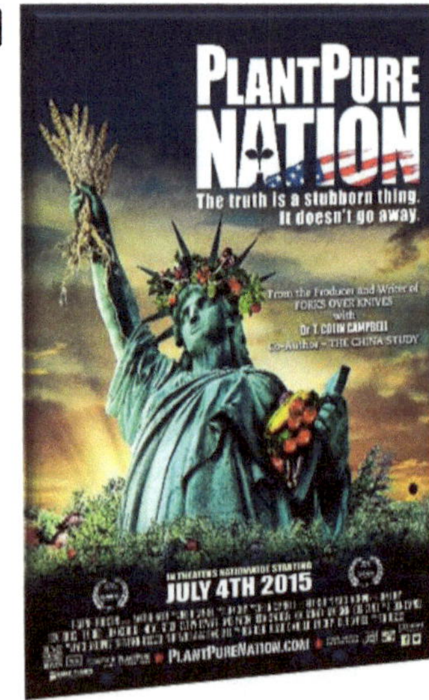

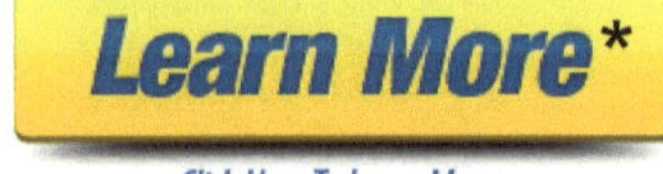

Click Here To Learn More...

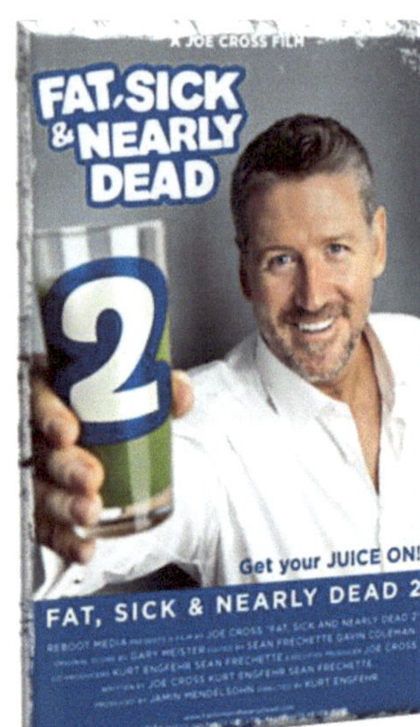

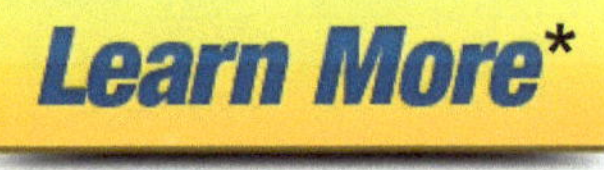

Click Here To Learn More...

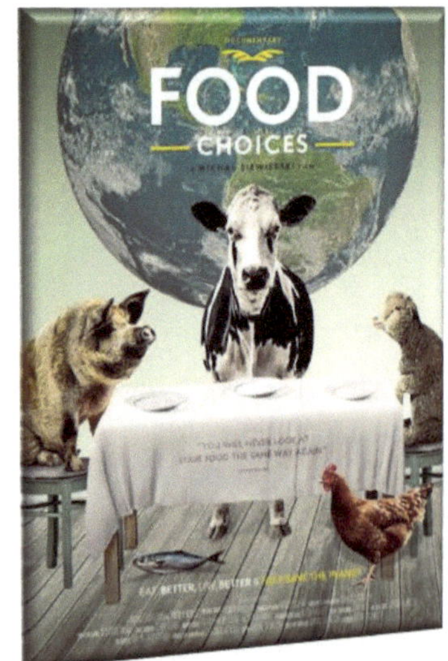

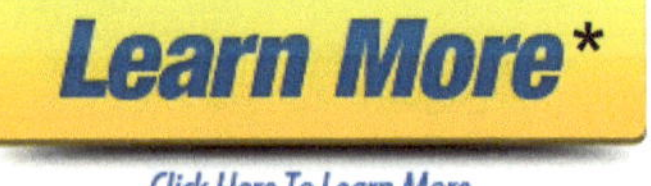

Click Here To Learn More...

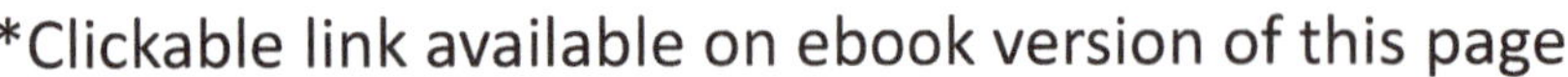

*Clickable link available on ebook version of this page

Documentaries To Watch

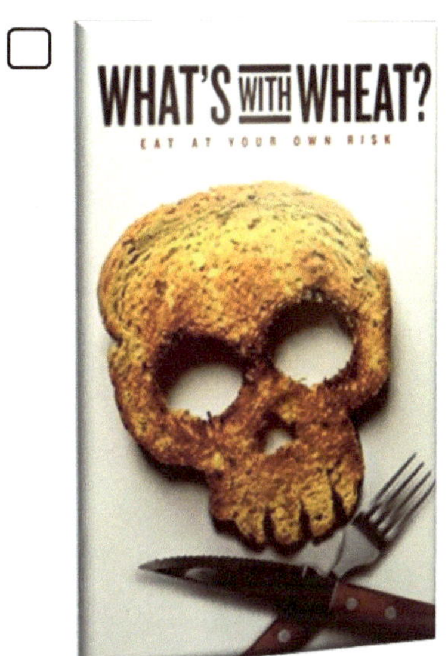

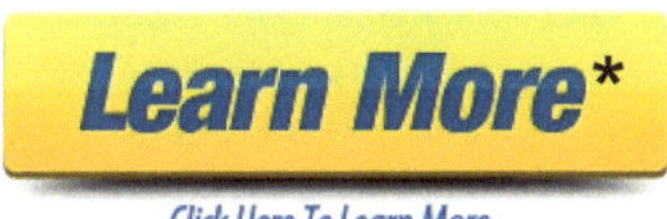

Click Here To Learn More...

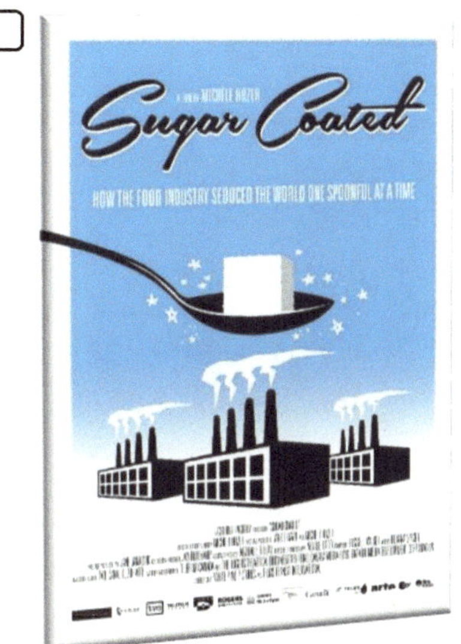

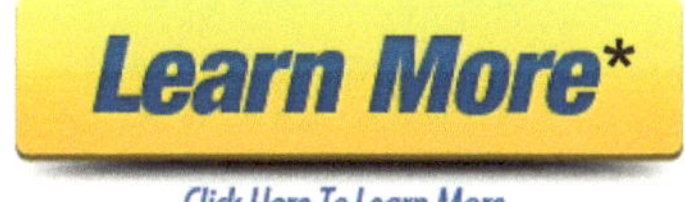

Click Here To Learn More...

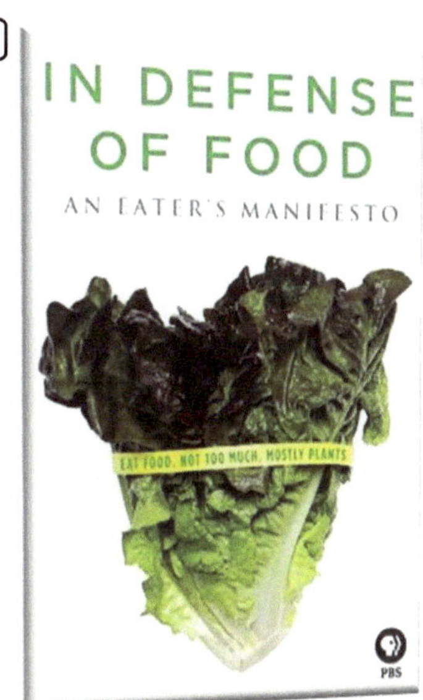

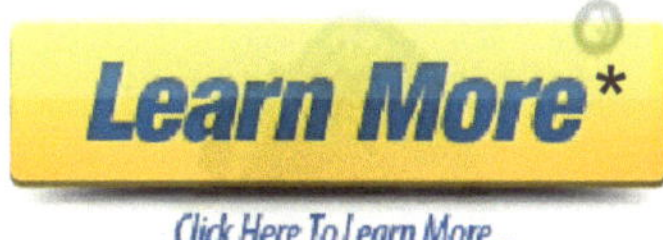

Click Here To Learn More...

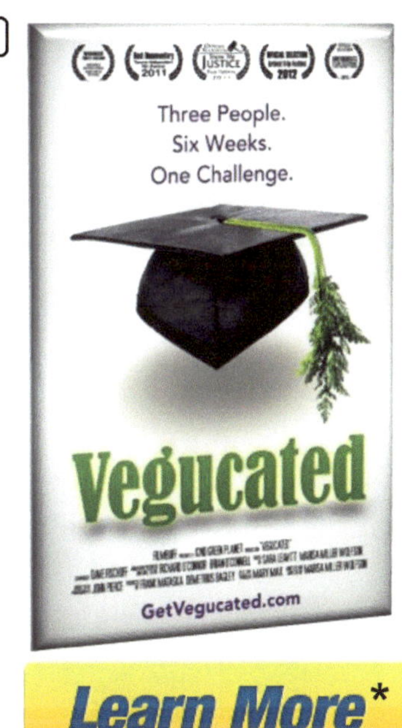

Learn More*

Click Here To Learn More...

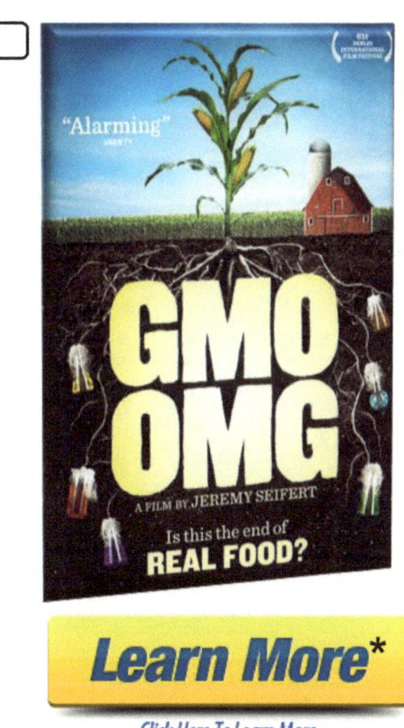

Learn More*

Click Here To Learn More...

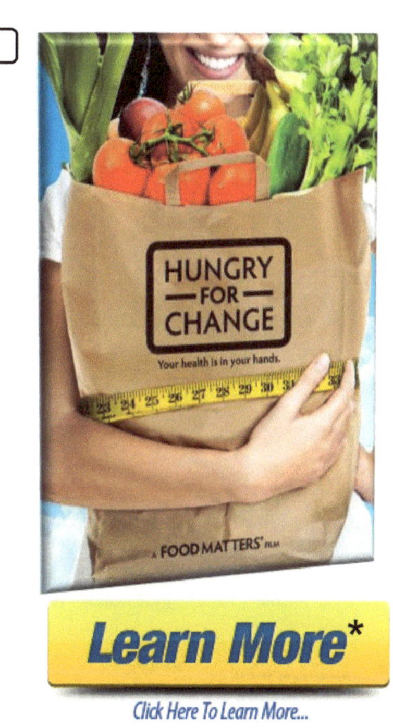

Learn More*

Click Here To Learn More...

*Clickable link available on ebook version of this page

Documentaries To Watch

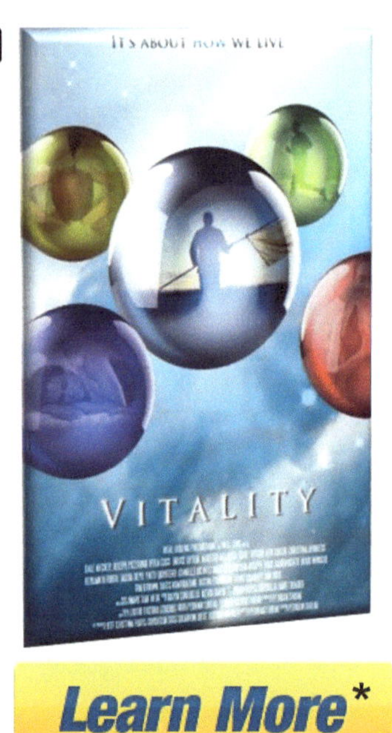

Learn More*

Click Here To Learn More...

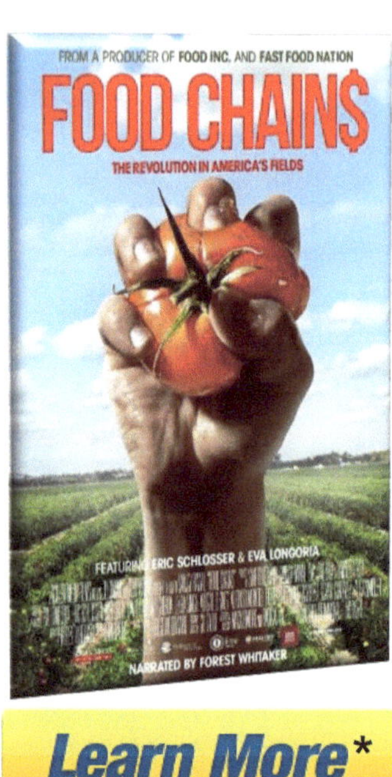

Learn More*

Click Here To Learn More...

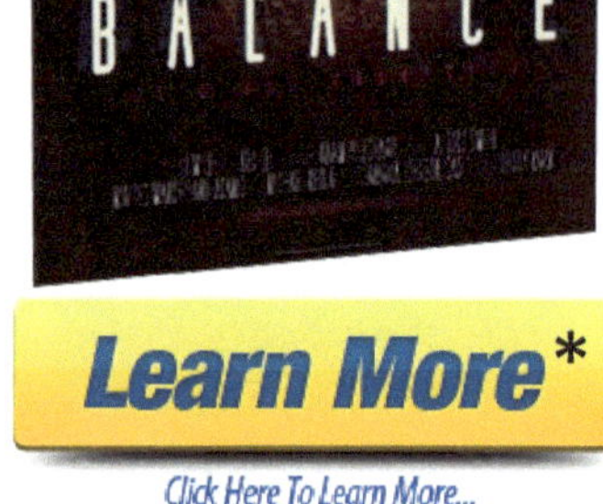

Learn More*

Click Here To Learn More...

Books To Read

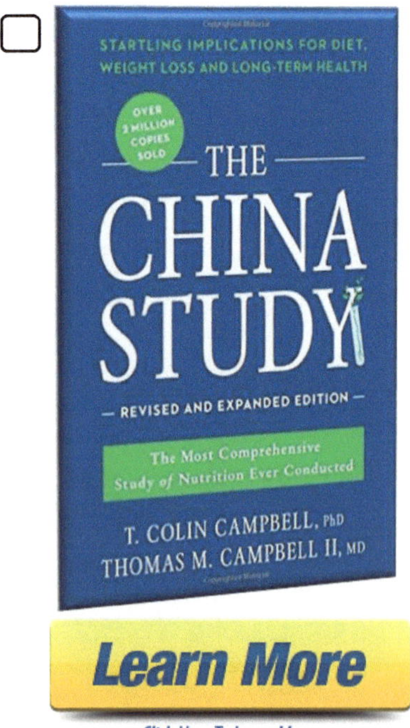

Learn More

Click Here To Learn More...

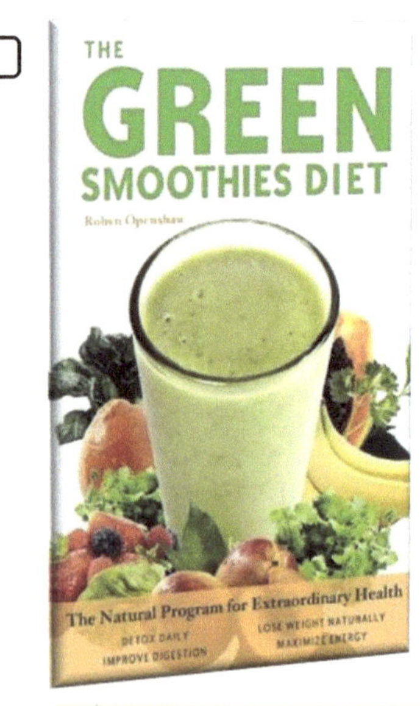

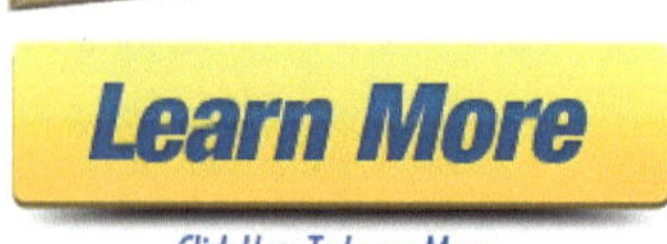

Learn More

Click Here To Learn More...

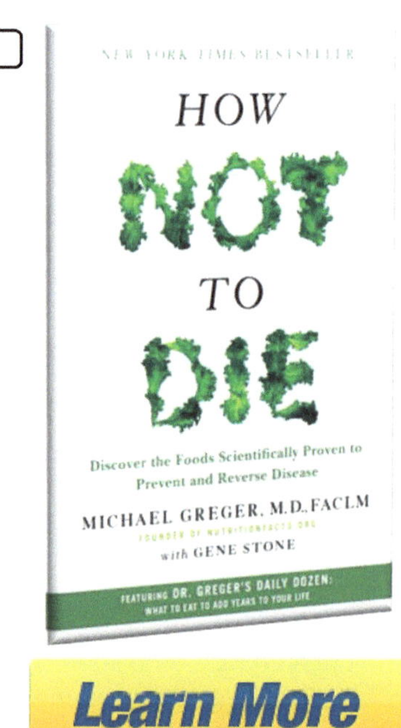

Learn More

Click Here To Learn More...

*Clickable link available on ebook version of this page

Summary

"Be the change that you wish to see in the world." - Mahatma Gandhi

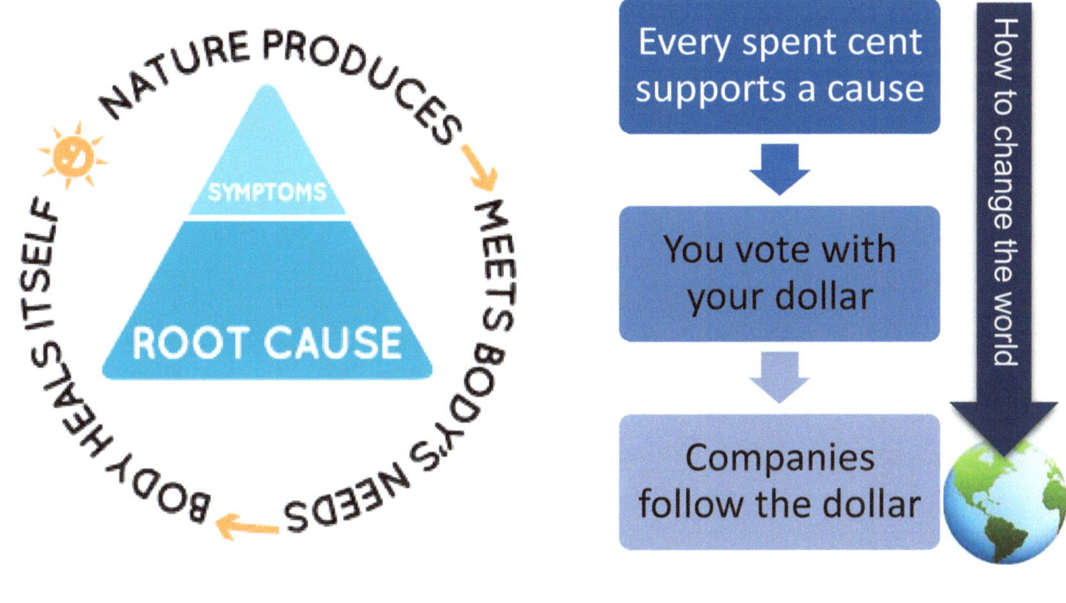

Top 10 Benefits Of 30 Day
Green Smoothie Challenge*

1.) 85% said… more energy
2.) 79.5% said… better digestion
3.) 50% said… weight loss
4.) Decrease heart disease risk
5.) Decrease cancer risk (See China Study)
6.) 10-15 minutes to make (Quick & Easy)
7.) 700% more nutrition than average American
8.) 10-15 servings of fruits and veggies
9.) 15 grams of extra fiber (Get regular!)
10.) 25 grams extra protein (Build lean muscle)

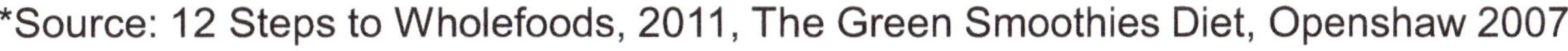

*Source: 12 Steps to Wholefoods, 2011, The Green Smoothies Diet, Openshaw 2007

Next Steps

1.) <u>Pro</u>: <u>Ongoing Support</u>	<u>Price</u>	<u>Special</u>
❑ 30 Days Coaching	~~9,997~~	4,997
❑ 60 Days Coaching	~~14,997~~	9,997
❑ 90 Days Coaching	~~19,997~~	14,997

2.) <u>Standard:</u> <u>One Time Support*</u>	<u>Price</u>	<u>Special</u>
❑ Las Vegas Strip Vegan Food Tour (2.5 hrs)	~~147~~	97
❑ SouthWest Vegan Food Tour (2.5 hrs)	~~147~~	97
❑ Chinatown Vegan Food Tour (2.5 hrs)	~~147~~	97
❑ In Home Pantry Review (1 hr)	~~127~~	97
❑ Let's Go Grocery Shopping (1 hr)	~~127~~	97
❑ In Home Breakfast Demo (2 hrs)	~~167~~	97
❑ In Home Lunch Demo (2 hrs)	~~167~~	97
❑ In Home Dinner Demo (2 hrs)	~~167~~	97
❑ Plant Powered Progress Book (Paperback)	~~20~~	15

Price per person

3.) <u>Start:</u> Follow & Learn

❑ Instagram: @tropicalsmoothieguy

4.) Contact Lance

- Email: thetropicalsmoothieguy@gmail.com
- Text: 214-906-0561

Scan with your phone camera below

5.) Visit https://linktr.ee/tropicalsmoothieguy to learn more

Lance's Story

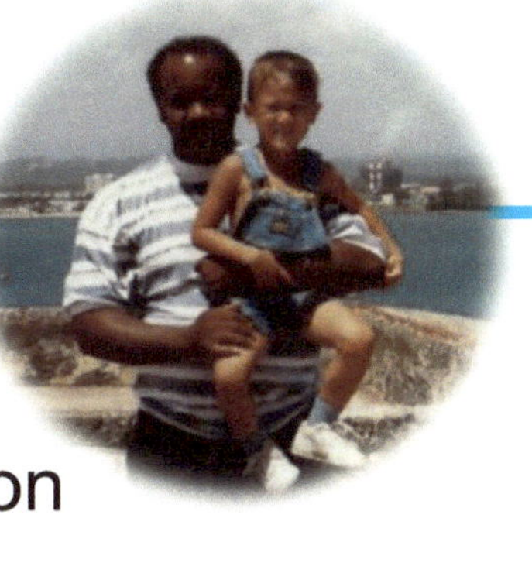

1997

Dad passed away from allergic reaction to Chemo & Throat Cancer

"My family health issues have given me an appreciation for my mind, body, and spirit." – Lance McGowan

2001

Mom's Triple Bypass Surgery & her medication use

2004

My Allergic Reaction to Tylenol 3 w/Codeine after breaking ankle doing hurdles

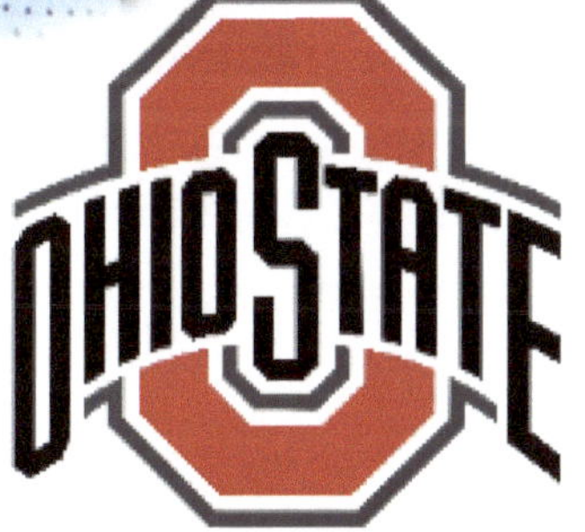

2004-2008

B.S. Marketing & Transportation (Columbus, OH)

PEPSICO
2008-2014

Analyst & Supervisor (Dallas, TX, Lynchburg, VA, Las Vegas, NV)

2013

Attended 1st Green Smoothie Class

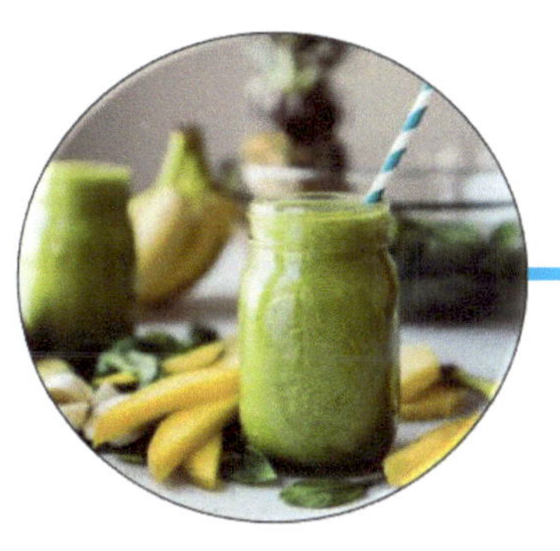

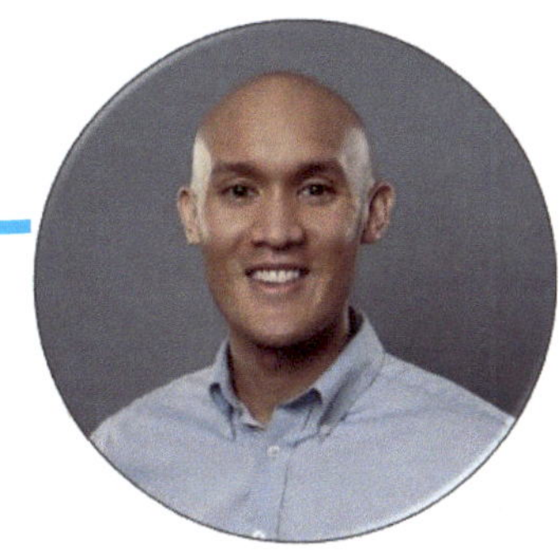

Today

Author, Speaker, Natural Solutions Educator (Las Vegas)

Lance's Story Cont...

My Mom's Story

I have many fond memories of my mom and I going out to eat together when I was growing up. She would often say that she would have a craving for a "Big Mac" or "Whopper" and I thought nothing of it and was just glad to spend time with her and get a free meal!

Over time, my mom started having trouble going up steps due to a shortness of breath. She started to take the elevator way more when the steps would have been her first choice before. She also was very adamant about living in a first story home in Columbus, Ohio and I never thought twice about it, but just wanted to support her decision.

After decades of the Standard American Diet (or SAD), my mom opted for triple bypass surgery in 2000 when I was 14 years old. I remember waiting outside of the hospital in Columbus, Ohio as I talked to my older sister who was smoking outside. She told me to keep her smoking habit a secret and I immediately knew that my sister was going down the same path as my mom. You see, my mom also used to smoke and she says she quit right after she was pregnant with me. Ironically enough, my sister is on more drugs than our mom and has a diminished quality of life too.

After my mom's triple bypass surgery, she got on prescription cholesterol and blood pressure medications. I saw my mom go from a healthy and energetic woman to a scarred up mom with diminished energy and a negative outlook on life. My mom's quality of life further deteriorated as she became more and more dependent on a pill for an ill and I felt powerless and misinformed as a young teenager.

At the time I was confused about what happened and wondered if my mom would be taken away from me. Fear of abandonment and separation anxiety was a normal part of my teenage life. I didn't know how she got into her situation at the time, but I knew that I didn't want anyone else to experience what I went through.

My Turning Point

I knew because I didn't have an MD behind my name, I didn't work in a fancy office, nor did I wear a white coat, that my mom would be less likely to take my advice. It wasn't until I went to a green smoothie class in Las Vegas in 2013 did everything change for me. I became fully independent with my healthcare from that day on and I became more passionate about helping people to improve their quality of life with natural solutions and a more whole foods lifestyle when they were ready for the education that was poured into me.

About Lance

Lance McGowan serves as the Chief Visionary Officer (CVO) of Eduvitae LLC and has helped thousands of people improve their health with natural solutions online and locally in Las Vegas.

Lance produces daily content online to add value to stay at home moms, employees, and entrepreneurs with Wellness Programs that reduce healthcare costs, improve quality of life, and reduce the risk of a premature death.

Lance holds a Bachelor's degree in Marketing and Transportation from the Ohio State University and has 6+ years of previous Corporate and Field based work experience at PepsiCo.

About Eduvitae LLC
Founded in 2014, eduvitae was built on the mission of sharing a more whole food lifestyle and natural solutions with people around the world. Having seen for himself the incredible benefits that can be had from using whole foods and plant based medicine, Lance McGowan set out to make this mission of helping 1 million people a reality. Eduvitae stands for "education is life" and empowering others is at the heart of everything the company stands for.

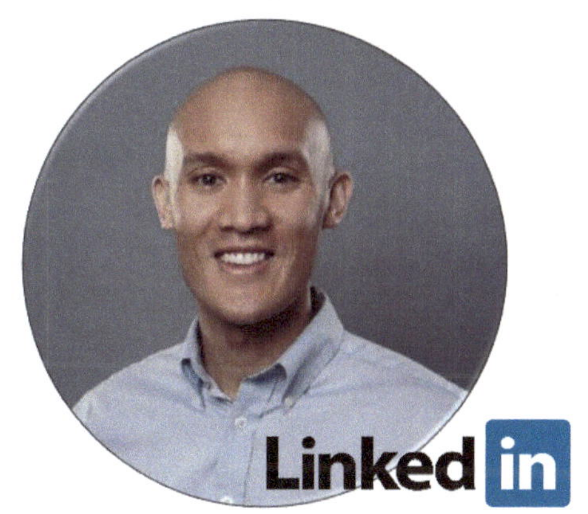